ASYLUM DAYS:
A Psychiatrist's Casebook

ASYLUM DAYS:

A Psychiatrist's Casebook

Peter J. Blockey

The Book Guild Ltd
Sussex, England

Although based on fact, the names and details of doctors and patients have been altered in this account in order to preserve confidentiality.

The Book Guild Ltd.
25 High Street,
Lewes, Sussex

First published 1996

Set in Times
Typesetting by Acorn Bookwork, Salisbury, Wiltshire

Printed in Great Britain by
Bookcraft (Bath) Ltd.

A catalogue record for this book is
available from the British Library

ISBN 1 85776 107 3

CONTENTS

For Corinne

and in memory of

Henry Yellowlees
Mary Mears
Jean Biggar
and James McPherson

who helped much more than they knew

PREFACE

When we landed at Chicago, I was (typically and characteristically) the last one off the aircraft. I joined a longish queue for inspection by the lone immigration officer; he was a squat individual clad in navy blue serge, and almost certainly armed. To a naive and slightly intimidated Englishman, he looked the very epitome of surly American officialdom. Eventually I handed him my passport, which he scrutinised thoughtfully.

At length he passed the document back to me.

'You a medical doctor?'

I conceded that I was.

'What kind of medicine you practise?'

'I'm a shrink. Mental work. A psychiatrist.' (Even at home, I habitually led up to this admission by a series of circumlocutions.)

His attitude had a curious solemnity, as of one who has mulled over all the implications and set a seal upon his judgement.

'That's the kind I like.' (Short pause.) 'You try to get to the bottom of things.'

I have never forgotten the pensive courtesy of that first encounter with an American on his native soil.

* * *

In the early years of this century, the doyen of British mathematicians was a man by the name of Hardy – and it is still a name to conjure with. It is said of him that towards the end of a long hour in the classroom, having covered all but a tiny space of the large blackboard, he was about to complete the penultimate line of his work when he uttered the words, 'It is now obvious...' and came to an abrupt halt. He paused for a moment and without more ado disappeared from the scene. A few minutes later he reappeared, no doubt a little dishevelled and breathless, and with a contented nod he said, 'Yes, it *is* obvious...' and filled in the last remaining tiny space at the bottom of the board.

* * *

Not very long ago, after another distinguished mathematician from our local university had given a public lecture, I was approached by another senior member of the mathematical fraternity, accompanied by his wife; I had as it happened recently attended a short series of evening classes which David was giving.

'Mary,' he said, 'this is Peter Blockey; he is, ah, he's a retired psychiatrist.' And his gaze sought my confirmation of this unlikely calling.

His wife, on the other hand, was enchanted. 'How much more exciting,' she suggested, 'than applied mathematics.'

It was nice of her to say so. I demurred as decorously as I could, and said that my vocation was truly a bizarre kind of discipline. I meant every word of it.

Hardy's dilemma – apocryphal as it may well be – could serve us well in illuminating the difficulties of our understanding, of our 'getting to the bottom of things' in the Western intellectual tradition. For however far we dig in the search for the origins of our being, we must always be left with sensible questions which are beyond proof or falsification, and we see only with hindsight how the impossibilities of yesterday have become the commonplace opportunities of today.

Consider the words of a psychoanalyst: 'All new challenges in life require a renegotiation of earlier tasks. If the new task can be successfully managed, the personality is further strengthened, but if earlier stages left too many defences unchanged, then the result is a breakdown...'[1]

I shall take it for granted that psychoanalysis, under certain very stringent and restrictive economic and psychological circumstances, can be incomparably beneficial. However, different schools take different stages of development as the locus of origin for our personal ('neurotic') difficulties; then again there appears to be no really uniform agreement among analysts as to how analysis works, nor yet as to what constitutes a sound 'analytic technique'. Even worse, one very distinguished practitioner (D W Winnicott) used the term 'corrective experience' to apply to situations which are valid and helpful within a psychoanalytic context, yet cannot be constructed to order, and should indeed in principle not be sought.

But first we must face up to the problem of the distracted mathematician, and withdraw a little in order to advance.

* * *

What makes people take up psychiatry?

Very well then, *how* do people come to take up psychiatry? Well, obviously enough, in various ways.

To begin with, hardly anyone takes to psychiatry as such because they are aware of their own needs ('have insight'). And most of those who do so will take psychiatry on board as a practical necessity before turning to some form of psychoanalysis, which requires its own brief comment at a later stage.

On the continent of Europe, psychiatry exists for the most part as an afterthought to the practice of 'neuropsychiatry' or of neurology – that is, of the medical approach to diseases of the nervous system. And there are some British workers who achieve distinction through the same route.

There are, also, occasional centres where psychiatry is taught with such verve that there is no other branch of medicine left to them which exerts so much appeal. (Is it not indeed the lot of the rare gifted teacher anywhere that he weave such an enchanted net as will ensnare his students to follow the same magic pathway?)

For the rest, I do not know. Accident and contingency no doubt play their part. But because the effort cost me and my family so much sweat, some hardship and some discomfort, I am duty bound to set out some of the nuts and bolts relative to the process.

I cannot think that anyone in his right mind would knowingly set out to embark upon a specialist career in full awareness of what is involved. A basic medical qualification in itself requires five or six years of unremitting toil; it is true some people seem to take it in their stride, and a few even follow up an existing qualification – in classics, say, or even in engineering – with a full medical training. But many thoroughly competent practitioners will still speak with awe and horror of the number of times some subject or other in the curriculum has defeated their attempts to master it. At my own last count there were 40 separate and distinct subjects to be taught and examined before one can so much as write a prescription – or make out a death certificate.

And it goes on. A capable individual in general practice may acquire fresh skills and qualifications into middle life, and continue to learn until at sixty-five or seventy he is too old to keep thoroughly up to date any more.

For an aspiring specialist the case is much much worse. The law requires at least one full year's work in two separate branches of the art before full registration. Many go on to posts of another full year or more to gain practical experience before embarking on middle-grade specialisation and committing themselves to whole-hearted study for a higher qualification – usually membership or a fellowship of an appropriate Royal College, whose examinations carry pass rates of about 12 per cent. The very brightest will take a second and sometimes even a third degree, and a few men succeed in acquiring higher qualifications in two or even (rarely) three different disciplines. Then another four years or more will follow at a senior level in the hope ultimately of acquiring a permanent post at top rank.

Of course there are those – the very brightest – who succeed without apparent effort in covering themselves with glory, and I have dwelt on matters in this tedious detail only to provide a framework and set the scene (mix thoroughly and add seasoning to taste) for the sketches which follow. The usual skulduggery, deceipt, politicking, diplomacy and pure bloody luck, to say nothing of well-deserved reward, are mostly omitted. Let's see how it goes.

1

Overture and Beginners

Six of us stepped out of the college doors on a February afternoon – the doors closed firmly behind us – to face a scene as uniformly grey as only that particular city can provide. The college (or as much of it as we had been allowed to see) was not an impressive building, for all its power and prestige. The street in which it lies is probably by now a busy thoroughfare for traffic from the south to the west of the city: at the time, it seemed to be saved from an air of dismal poverty only because it lies near the edge of an area of wide Georgian terraces and parks, and within easy reach of the centre of one of the more extraordinary cities in Europe.

One of us had a camera, and we stood briefly together for a snapshot before dispersing. Each of us clutched a vast document in Latin. There were no celebrations: we all had homes to go to and jobs to find, though first we had each of us, separately and severally, to make our way to another of the Royal Colleges in order to sign a big, black, brass-bound book. These two colleges, together with a third, 45 miles to the west, were empowered to confer licences which entitled registration with the General Medical Council, and a great many eminent refugees had qualified all over again in order to obtain the modest 'TQ' (Triple Qualification) which would allow them to ply their trade in the strange grey kingdom so effectively cut off from the rest of Europe. One of us indeed was such a man; older than the rest of us, a Lithuanian. I have often marvelled at the courage of those who grappled with a taxing curriculum in such a strange language in order to survive, and I wonder what *did* happen to him.

Fortunately, from now on, I knew some of the drill, and I struck lucky at my first attempt. My last clinical tutor and mentor had a position at the Royal Institution which I mistakenly believed to carry the kind of rank which would allow him to take me on as a houseman. He was a civilised man with a firm grasp of surgical principles. Unknown to me, and as luck would have it, he had just secured his first consultancy at a little hospital down the road, and I fancy he was a little startled to be approached by an ignorant and diffident volunteer at precisely the moment when he needed a very junior pair of hands. His position at the Royal Institution was in truth an unenviable one. In those days it had been described as 'a series of cottage hospitals, inefficiently run'. The fact is that only those who were prepared to wait for dead men's shoes, rather than submit to the indignity of earning a very honest surgical penny in some provincial centre, could have any hope of reaching the top in the Institution.

Alec Sutherland was one such, and he had grafted for years under a chief whose competence was long past its best, coping manfully with the surgical bread and butter of piles, varicose veins and hernias, and accepting at least one night each week the commitment to take on board anything and everything that emergency surgery could throw at him. He bore his lot manfully: he was invariably patient and uncomplaining, sustaining his work at a steady pace, without hurry and without fuss. Partly, I think, he genuinely enjoyed his work; certainly he displayed a uniformly workmanlike surgical craftsmanship, and his knowledge of surgery was wide-ranging and far-sighted. At all events, his patience bore fruit in the end, for once he was established, it was rumoured that he enjoyed the largest private practice in the city, and this in a centre whose surgical traditions spanned four or five centuries and the whole width of Europe.

His first consultancy, and my own first professional post, was at a small hospital on the edge of the city, which enjoyed loyal support from the local community which it had served from Victorian times through to the great economic depression of the thirties and beyond. The community itself had long since been swallowed up administratively into the city, but the hospital never deteriorated into one of the vast specialised units scattered over ten miles or more of urban gloom or sylvan and inaccessible limits spread around the periphery of the great centre itself: it continued to provide local services to local people and to enjoy local pride and local loyalties in the same tradition which it had always had. And it showed.

From the very start, Alec's own unit ran as if on oiled wheels. His theatre sister, Katie Ashe, was a comely and totally capable young woman who tackled everything with thoroughgoing competence and goodwill. Alec himself invariably worked at the same steady pace, neither fussing and fiddling nor cutting a dash with the speed of his ectomies. Anaesthetists were invariably prompt and (marvellous to relate) we were spared any of the icy silences or vicious barbs which can be commonplace between the mighty experts at opposite ends of the sleeping subject of their endeavours.

Katie eyed me as a potential menace for a few moments after my first entry on stage. She tried me out sharply with a question on size of glove, which I parried superbly with an assumed air of nonchalance by giving her a size which was not in stock. With a fine display of casual machismo I proceeded to snap the appropriate article sharply over the folded surgical gown at the wrist. The glove tore, and at the third attempt, Katie, with genuine kindness, gently suggested that surgical gloves had a measurable cash value and would respond better to a more delicate approach. They did, and Katie (who was in reality always very properly addressed by title) thereafter consistently proved to be a fount of essential wisdom in all matters surgical.

'You will find,' she said, 'that it is easier to stand at the table if you take part of the weight by leaning against it with your iliac crests.' I tried this too, and it worked. Except that Katie, in her kindness, had used the term 'iliac crests' when she meant (*quelle délicatesse*) 'junction of the pubic bones'.

And to this day, I still pick up a pair of scissors between

thumb and middle finger because, that way, one can swing the scissors round against the sleeve and keep them ready for use to cut stitches as the master puts them in. And then the index finger is ready to prise the instrument loose from the digits which it so awkwardly embraces, with decisive speed and precision.

For the most part, Alec's patients throve as they deserved to do in the hands of his loyal and experienced team. One who did not nevertheless helped to teach me a lesson in the value of simple remedies diligently applied.

It came about that we admitted a man for partial removal of the stomach – a major piece of surgery in anybody's hands. When I came to take his history, I could make nothing of it at all; there was no choice but to rely on the chief's experience and expertise, and within a day or two, a partial gastrectomy was duly carried out. So far, so good. A little later, as I made my way towards the far end of the ward, a young lady followed me in and lightly leapt upon the central row of lockers which were a feature of the solid interiors of that day. The first I knew of this was a string of instructions worthy of a sergeant-major: the young lady was a physiotherapist – one of a breed not to be taken lightly. She was there to conduct post-operative breathing exercises for the entire ward, and for a moment I nearly snapped to attention, thumbs neatly along the trouser seams, and joined in.

This time, however, all was not well, though this was not apparent until some days later, when the ward sister gently murmured that the gentleman with the gastrectomy appeared to be oozing blood-stained fluid – a sign of imminent rupture of the sutures. Since her advice was not of a kind which brooked any delay, Alec himself was duly approached and proceeded to explore the situation. There was little to be done. A raging infection had spread everywhere. We removed as much as we could, and fresh firm sutures were applied round massive dressings. All was to no avail, and the hapless man slipped away from us despite all we could do.

Afterwards, it seemed clear that he must have been schizophrenic from the start, to account for his inability to give an adequate history, his inability to respond to the few clear simple commands of the 'physio', and his failure to complain or to show any sign of the raging infection which gripped him. But looking back, what I remember now is the salutary shock to self-esteem when everything has been done which could be done, only to leave behind a pathetic shambles of total defeat.

Alec's ward had its fair share of psychiatric features as a matter of course, and the most dire threat that his ward sister could offer in order to bring a recalcitrant patient into line was (in her own ears) the dreaded ultimatum of 'I will get the psychiatrist to you.' Once, indeed, she did so. No great harm came of it, and perhaps for my part even some good came from the encounter, though that, as they say, is another story.

Alec was a shrewd judge of company, and his words were well measured to any occasion. Once or twice he inadvertently let his feelings show, and one such occasion befell in the case of a man I remember simply as 'Ken'. To help to get Ken's condition in perspective calls for a certain perambulation round the mulberry bush, and this is not a temptation I am known to resist.

It came about much in this wise: Alec's patients may have displayed their fair share of psychiatric curiosities, while he, the chief himself, could not unfairly be portrayed as being the very model of a modern surgeon general. But Alec had opposite numbers. One was his assistant surgeon, who had his own idiosyncrasies. The other was a second chief in his own right, an independent being of a character so different as to verge on the alien. The two of them in fact rubbed along very well together when they had to, as befitted two senior fellows of the same learned college. Yet Hamish Robson had a character which almost beggared description. One had to know him – even briefly – in order to understand him. Physically, he was a big man, with a presence which made itself felt without yet quite achieving a Presence. And he does make for a big mulberry bush.

He had something of the character of a ballroom crystal, which illuminated now one facet and then in a moment some other quite unpredictable aspect. No one word ever quite fitted him. He was not incompetent, but nor did he have the uniformly high standard of craftsmanship which my own chief displayed. He was something of a buffoon, yet his abilities commanded a certain curious respect; while his name was a byword among those who knew him, he was not one (like the hospital's elderly physician) who had to be constantly protected from his own folly. He could be irascible, yet he could display a certain pompous joviality. His junior staff on the whole kept their distance, and he was invariably addressed as 'Sir', or by his full name, even in the cordial atmosphere of the junior mess.

He once terrorised his staff for three weeks on end by openly contemplating a total removal of the pancreas in a terminally ill woman. Such a heroic measure would, I think, have required teams of highly specialised surgeons working in relays, but this did not prevent him from openly carrying round a vast American monograph on the subject, which he used to deposit in the ante-room to the theatre. Only Sister Ashe remained detached.

The dreaded day dawned. There were, as I remember, four or five of us round the table, and Hamish duly made a small incision and explored the cavity with one finger. He duly pronounced his verdict – 'It's malignant' (more accurately, 'It's inoperable'). Each of us, in order of rank, was required to verify his opinion, Sister Ashe included, and myself, not yet one month qualified, last of all. With a suitably solemn countenance, and after a proper delay (during which I felt precisely nothing at all), I too gave my assent. The lady was allowed to slip away peacefully, and the rest of us to breathe more easily. Katie emerged with more credit than the rest of us: her fears were for the patient, and not for herself.

On another occasion, Hamish was concluding a short and straightforward repair of the abdominal wall – a ventral hernia – in the company of his own houseman, who was an elegant, upright, well-spoken young man from a good public school. He was known, as it happens, by the name of 'Mak', being remotely of Greek origin, with a family name something like Makarios Theotocopoulos. At all events, Mr Robson Sir was in the process of closing the wound by passing a series of straight needles neatly in a row through the skin margins, leaving Mak to pull them through and tie off the threads. Sir was in expansive mood, and confided jovially to his young assistant, 'You know, me boy, this is one of the most uniformly gratifying operations to perform ... invariably excellent results ... always radical cure...' and more of the like. Then one of his needles punctured a vein, a little vein, invisible to the eye, and the tiny pristine field of operation filled inexorably with an expanding pool of dark blood. The flow of words darkened, uninterrupted, along with the gentle flow of blood – 'God damn and blast it, why does this always happen to me?' Gentle pressure with a gauze swab soon staunched the flow of words and blood alike, and the operation concluded in peace – and in silence.

Finally, within the few days before my temporary attachment to Sir came to an end, Hamish undertook to remove a chronically infected area from the edge of a shin bone. When we were all assembled and awaiting the entrance of the star turn, Sister let it be known in her own soft conspiratorial way that Mr R would be needing the drill, but since he had not asked for it, no preparations had been made for its use. The drill, in fact, turned out to be an ordinary electric household affair equipped with a hinged chromium casing which could be sterilised to make it suitable for use at the table. The operation was straightforward enough, but it concluded for some reason with the need to pass a piece of stout material – 'kangaroo tendon' – through the sharp edge of the shin bone just beneath the skin. Accordingly, the following conversation ensued:

'I'll take the drill now, Sister.'

'The drill, Mr Robson?'

'Yes, yes, the drill, Sister, the drill.'

'But you didn't ask for the drill, Mr Robson.'

Hamish was over a barrel, and he knew it.

For a while, his perplexed exasperation was almost tangible in face of the silent expectancy of his team.

What followed was a tribute as much to the dedication of

surgical instrument makers as to Hamish's capacity for inept extemporisation. For in his desperation he seized upon a pair of towel clips and applied them to the sharp front edge of the shin bone. And then he wiggled them about.

Now towel clips are designed to attach sterile towels around those areas of skin which do not need to be exposed at operation (skin cannot be completely sterilised, and most of the patient must remain covered if for no other reason than to preserve body heat). So the ends of the clips are made as sharp as they well can be, in order to penetrate with the least possible harm, and for the same reason they are also made of the softest reasonable material. So when Hamish attacked bone with sharp instruments scrupulously designed to penetrate textile and to spare living tissue, they did what they were very carefully intended to do – they simply curled up and died. Hamish was not one to hurl things around the theatre, and Sister must have laid her plans with care, because sterile metal covers for the drill appeared in time to prevent any further wanton sacrifice of costly instruments.

Hamish, then, could be, and often was, a thoroughly petulant individual. Consequently it did nothing for his equanimity when a troop of top-flight American surgeons descended upon the local college. I heard him chuntering away about it one morning over coffee with Alec. He was thoroughly discomfited, and clearly felt that transatlantic surgery was a discipline in an altogether different field, of almost extraterrestrial sophistication.

Alec was not to be drawn, and made some noncommital remark in his own dismissive way, concealing his own misgivings with a veneer of well-merited aplomb – 'Oh, I think we could still teach them a thing or two' – or something of that kind. The consequences were none the less distinctly interesting.

Hamish's response was pretty prompt and brutal, for it happened that higher examinations for fellowship of the college were under way, and I learned something of the manner in which examinations can be conducted.

Again, I caught a whisper of it over coffee the following

morning. Hamish had scrupulously threaded his way through the minefield of unspoken conventions which led to seniority in his profession, and consequently had achieved the august status of an examiner. It was therefore his privilege to consult the relevant literature (most of which he must surely have forgotten) and to find some fragment of arcane learning with which he could hope to skewer his candidates' laboriously acquired inventory of useless knowledge, and their perilously fragile morale, all at a single stroke. I heard him boasting of this technique more than once.

But Alec's reaction was more measured, more considered, and more to be savoured.

It came about in this wise: the physicians of the hospital had undertaken the care of a middle-aged working man for whom they had requested a surgical opinion. This was Kenneth, who had an unusual history.

Ken had little by little begun to reject his food – physically, and not in the least because of any quirk in his psychology. It turned out that for a good many months he had been unable to retain any solids at all, and precious little by way of liquid. He had, moreover, steadfastly refused to consider admission to hospital, until the point was reached at which his level of undernourishment was so profound as to leave him in the throes of a delirium which made his admission imperative and undeniable. He was by this stage profoundly anaemic, and the physicians ('magicians') set to work to determine the nature and degree of his anaemia, to administer the appropriate remedies and day by day to measure their effect (if any) upon his parlous state. Alec, possibly reluctant to meddle with undue haste in such an unpromising predicament, bided his time until, as it happened, the American surgeons were on the point of embarking upon a full-scale formal dinner with the surgical luminaries of the city. Before the evening began, Alec rang me up.

'How's that man on the medical ward, Blockey?... Well find out, and I'll ring you back later.'

After dinner he did ring back. I told him that the junior physician had reported that Kenneth's haemoglobin was evidently approaching – very slowly – about one-third of the value it should have had.

Alec snorted. 'That man's dying. Blockey, while the magicians sit there and fiddle.'

There was no answer to that one, and no need of an answer. Alec filled the gap himself.

'I'm coming in, Blockey.'

And so it came about that towards eleven o'clock, Alec sat in the quiet dim-lit medical ward for all the world like Rodin's *Thinker*, assuming a very fair portrayal of a great surgeon on the brink of a life-and-death decision. He timed his long pause for reflection really very well, and at length looked me full in the face.

Solemn, brisk and decisive, he declared emphatically, 'We've got to go in.'

Towards midnight we gathered round Kenneth's inert body on the table. As he stood with knife poised. Alec confided, almost conspiratorially, 'Of course it's malignant; but we do have to have a look.'

Accordingly, he made a keyhole incision, through which his experienced right index finger disappeared into Kenneth's abdomen – much after the fashion which Hamish had done a few weeks before.

This time the result was far different. After a very short time, the atmosphere was electrified: (it has always seemed to me entirely appropriate that on this side of the Atlantic, the operating room should be given the term 'theatre').

Alec's opening line was simply, 'Good God, me boy, it's benign.'

Much as before, I too was bidden to verify the finding. And sure enough, my own inexpert and inexperienced finger found a smooth, round, firm, elastic, mobile lump, clearly due to fibrous scarring, and not the hard, irregular, fixed mass of a cancer.

Alec was in his element. The incision was enlarged and in the next two or three hours the obstruction at the exit of Kenneth's stomach was bypassed, creating a passage directly from the stomach into the small bowel; a gastro-enterostomy which would allow adequate nourishment to pass once again freely into the gut. Only once, about half past two in the morning, Alec allowed himself a moment's exasperation with Jim Cooper, the trainee who had come along to be helpful, but before three o'clock he was back at the seat of his stylish sports saloon and on his way home, honour and confidence restored.

The next morning, Ward Sister (Surgical) summoned all her available staff to bear witness to the appalling physical condition that Kenneth was in. Months of effective starvation combined with substantial immobility had combined to give the poor man bedsores, which I am sure none of us could have anticipated even had we had several lifetimes in practice. Where a pad of fat should have cushioned the base of his spine, the skin had been broken over an area the size of a large soup-plate, and only a thick wodge of blackened necrotic tissue concealed the naked bone of his sacrum from our horrified gaze. His heels and elbows were similarly afflicted. Sister called us all to witness that these dreadful lesions were present on admission to her ward. Within the hour, Sister Medical had announced firmly that his sores had not appeared under her care. The medical staff concluded that they must have appeared on the trolley bearing him from the medical ward to the theatre.

Meanwhile, his delirium shattered the peace of the acute surgical ward. He had what is known as an 'occupational delirium', and as he had been a foreman at the local docks, this consisted of bawling alternatively into the depths of an imaginary ship's hold, and then upwards to an equivalent height towards an equally imaginary crane-driver. Patients and staff alike bore this performance with unbelievable fortitude, but the fifth morning saw a change.

I began my round that day on the opposite side of the ward, and when I drew level with Kenneth's bed, he motioned me across to his side of the ward. His face bore a faintly puzzled air, and he asked me in the most moderate way, and with complete good sense, how long he had been where he was. I told him, and he persisted, 'Yes, but was I somewhere else before I came here?'

I confirmed that he had spent three weeks in another ward of the same hospital. He looked relieved, and a little pensive. Then, combining hesitation with urgency in the same request, he asked had he perhaps been, well, not quite right in the head. I told him gently that indeed he had had a period of some disturbance. His relief was transparent, and he settled back in his bed more comfortably, knowing that his mangled memories of the last few weeks were not just some malignant unreality of his imagination.

On Alec's next visit to the ward, he was almost jubilant. He was well aware of my own aspirations, and of my shortcomings as a surgical handyman, but his pragmatic Scottish magnanimity accommodated both, and with the merest hint of complacency he remarked, 'There you are, me boy; that's psychiatry for you.'

In Alec's world, surgery was as uniformly successful as psychiatry was futile. I could believe even today that there was some justice in his faith.

What surprises me still is that four days on a liquid diet should have been enough to restore Kenneth's equilibrium to normal. His change was so profound and his intake so little that the effect seemed little short of miraculous.

Kenneth's physical condition was less responsive, and when my contract expired some months later, there was still little sign of substantial healing in the ghastly space where healthy tissue should have been. To this day, I cannot imagine what measures could have been taken to restore the terrible damage which Kenneth had unwittingly inflicted upon himself. But the transformation in a matter of days from raving confusion to complete lucidity was, with one exception, as dramatic as anything I have met beyond the realms of fiction.

* * *

When my term was completed, I was as fortunate in my next post as I had been in the first. I had chanced upon the notice of a vacancy for a junior hand in a university department of psychiatry within striking distance alike of my home and the training school where I had spent so many enlightening years.

I have always believed that the notice had been circulated by hand around the medical schools of the country before reaching the usual journals, since my enquiry drew a gratifyingly prompt response and an almost immediate interview. I remember this with some pleasure, not least because of the part which Alec had played in his support.

Alec had known full well that my choice of work as his own first junior was one which was forced upon me by the regulations of the day, and when I approached him on the matter of a reference, he agreed cordially enough, asking me to return the next day. This I did; he confirmed that a reference had been sent, and handed me a copy in a sealed brown envelope.

'It is short,' he said, in his own curiously economical way, 'but you will find it is enough.'

It was indeed: he had confirmed that I had worked for him for six months, that I had been diligent in my duties and that I had been courteous and agreeable in my dealings with patients and staff alike.

He could not have said, and did not say, that I showed any particular aptitude or zeal for the art of surgery, but when I faced the professor, he nodded in a solemn way at the scrap of paper which Alec had sent him, not knowing that I was aware of its contents, and remarked, 'That is a very good reference.'

Alex, of course, had been right, and I was later to learn more than once that it is often pleasanter to have colleagues who are agreeable rather than shrewdly, politically, ambitious and successful.

There was a hiatus of six weeks before I took up my new post, a gap which was eventful enough to alter the rest of my life and my family's life for a generation to come: the immediate effect was that I left my wife on a dark and stormy night and set forth in an ancient rattletrap across a hundred miles of moorland to join my new colleagues.

The unit was a small one, housed in a modern purpose-built ward set in open country, miles from the main teaching centre in the city where the professor himself held sway. We had a couple of dozen beds, and some occasional light duties in the large traditional hospital nearby. There were three medical staff in all on the observation ward, including Gordon, a middle-grade trainee, the registrar and Trudy, his senior, who answered to the most senior staff of all at the centre itself. Our duties were to care for those few patients who could either be guaranteed to recover with a short course of treatment, or whose condition was mysterious and required further investigation. Once a week we were visited by the professor himself, and one morning each week we visited the main department for demonstrations or discussions at the highest level.

The work in this setting was always fascinating, and the opportunities for exchange of views turned out to be quite intoxicating.

Gordon and Trudy were both thoroughly congenial, and so indeed was the atmosphere at the centre itself.

The professor himself had some of the qualities of Hamish Robson: unpredictable, larger than life, and capable of such indiscretions that a sort of conspiracy grew up among his staff of speaking in hints and whispers. He had a sad reputation for treachery; for myself, I found this reputation persistently grievous. All of us had good cause to be grateful to the man in one way or another, if only because of the highly colourful sense of drama which he presented on every occasion. In truth, it was only necessary to have a metaphorical salt-cellar available at all times, and all of us in the department constantly cast pinches of salt as a matter of course.

But it seems that one young man had been encouraged to spend a year abroad at a prestigious centre of learning with the juicy promise of substantial promotion on his return, only to be met 12 months later with a cheery greeting and a baldly innocent enquiry as to where he had been, and a 'What are you going to do next?'

It's the sort of thing which happens in almost any large organisation, usually perhaps with a little more subtlety. For my own part, I was in the fortunate position of being quite competent enough as well as much too junior to present any kind of problem, so that when our paths crossed, the professor could afford to be affable, which he managed in the most informal way without any obvious trace of condescension or patronage.

Trudy had independent means and was in any case married to a bright star in a different department, and she relished a greater freedom to voice her opinion than anyone else. The most senior staff, after the professor, were assured of permanent positions elsewhere sooner or later, and went their own way regardless. Two people were unequivocally loyal. They were the senior departmental nurse, Sister French, and the professor's own second in command, Dr Round. Neither had any aspirations elsewhere, and both quietly got on with their work, without any of the slightly frenzied chatter of higher examinations, publications or other prerequisites of promotion. It was almost as though we all pursued our paths in orbit around a massively luminous body, occasionally perturbing each other a little, with scarcely any effect on the dazzling star round whom we moved, and who pursued his own path in regions we could scarcely guess at.

Towards the end of my time there, the professor gave a sort of midsummer party to end all parties, and before we all wove our festively drunken way long after midnight around the periphery of the hospital to creep out by the back entrance, someone took a picture which seemed to embody the situation perfectly. The professor stood behind Sister French and Dr Round, each of them nearly a foot shorter than the chief, his arms cast around their shoulders in an entirely spontaneous and unaffected gesture of affection. He sported a discreet emblem of military distinction which he had gained in his own unorthodox way.

The three comrades in arms seemed to symbolise perfectly my own experience of six months memorably spent in an atmosphere of cordial goodwill and heady intellectual endeavour.

As for the shop floor, it has to be remembered that a psychiatrist's bread and butter, if not his staple diet, consisted at this time of long-term care for seriously disturbed individuals. At its best, this care could be of a very high standard, as when a body of wealthy Quakers set up a small private asylum for other Quakers towards the end of the eighteenth century. These Friends established a moral code which (with others) served as an ideal for nearly a hundred years. However, side by side with genuinely charitable intentions and some indisputable advances in humane care, it was publicly recognised at the beginning of the nineteenth century that conditions of extreme degradation occurred. After 1845 an Act of Parliament – with the best of intentions – provided for the compulsory erection for public asylums by each county in England. Inevitably, these became crowded, and with no systematically effective remedies available, standards varied from very bad, even atrocious, up to remarkably good – most notably perhaps in institutions which had been privately funded as charitable foundations, but which provided for the admission of pauper lunatics at a charge agreed with the parishes they served – in this case, in Scotland.

Even in the best establishments, however, there were physical conditions which condemned people to lingering death. About one in every seven people admitted for psychiatric care suffered from syphilitic infection of the brain, and until the advent of penicillin, only a minority of these responded to treatment. Again, schizophrenic patients were susceptible to pulmonary tuberculosis, for which there was no uniformly effective treatment until the introduction of streptomycin. I remember once or twice visiting a series of dark side-rooms, each containing a mute immobile figure, isolated and wasting away with the dreadful white plague.

At about the same time that penicillin and streptomycin became available, a safe and effective remedy for some varieties of depression also became generally available and widely used, but the need for long-term care on a large scale persisted. A few gifted psychiatrists either inherited or created a tradition of nursing care which achieved remarkably high standards, but in parts of the country standards were so oppressive that one senior psychiatrist whom I met refused to acknowledge the existence of his long-stay wards even after powerful and useful drugs came into use for the relief and management of the 'psychoses' (embracing severely disturbed behaviour, or in the plainest English, 'insanity').

There remained a number of people with 'nervous breakdown' or in the language of textbooks, 'neurosis'. 'Psychosis' and 'neurosis' deserve the comment that both are merely classical equivalents to 'condition of the mind' or 'condition of the nerves', both terms being designed to dignify ignorance by the use of jargon of archaic origin. In religious use, this practice is usual and acceptable; scientists also like their alpha rays, gamma rays, omega particles and the rest, and mathematicians their beta functions, zeta functions and the whole run of the Greek alphabet. Returning to our muttons, psychiatrists who aspired to clarity of definition quoted the German literature to the effect that a neurosis has symptoms which can be understood in 'rational' terms, while the psychoses do not, and require a special vocabulary to describe them.

The ultimate point of this digression is that neurotic patients – people with personal difficulties sufficiently severe to drive them to a psychiatrist – would be treated by the light of nature: that is to say, according to the personal inclination of the therapist. Psychoanalysis at this juncture is simply not (as a rule) a viable proposition, for severely practical reasons. Psychologists believing that what cannot be measured does not exist have been known to declare that 'the natural history of neurosis is towards spontaneous remission' – or more simply, serious personal difficulties clear up on their own with time. Experience suggests that neither the spontaneous responses of another individual, nor yet the mere passage of time, and not even the seductive and arcane theories of psychoanalysis, are adequate to cope with the realities. (The work of experimental and clinical psychologists had not been developed at this time; their contribution is growing and it will be interesting to see what comes of it.)

The mysteries of both neurotic and psychotic responses to management first made an impact on my own experience in the history of a young man called Ted.

* * *

Ted was a historian. My meeting with him must have been fortuitous, since Ted came under Gordon's care, and my regular duties confined me to the other half of the unit; the womenfolk came under Trudy's supervision. (It has to be borne in mind that in those days mixed-sex wards were unheard of.)

Something about Ted's bearing must have drawn me to him; he was perhaps more alert, more attentive to his surroundings than the usual mix of individuals, but at all events, I quickly discovered that he had an extensive knowledge of and a passion for military history. In anybody else this could have amounted to a monomania of monumental and pathological proportions, yet Ted possessed such a balanced and well-modulated manner of expressing himself that we were able to pursue one of the most fascinating conversations that I can recall. We lit on the topic of the Colt revolver. Ted knew each model by number, by date of introduction, by its defects, its ultimate success as 'the widowmaker', by its failings in further development and by its place and importance in relation to American history.

Then he went on to the Gatling gun, the ingenious early machine-gun, and with the same immaculate precision he summed up its dates, its manufacture and its ultimate failure.

Ted, it seemed, had set out to encompass his own end in the middle of winter by marching north (like the Roman Ninth Legion) until he simply disappeared from all further ken. He landed up at Brora, north of Inverness, having apparently covered more than 300 miles over some of the most inhospitable territory in Britain. Near Brora, some motorists, more or less by chance, happened to catch sight of him and came to the conclusion (not surprisingly) that there was something untoward about his behaviour. The upshot was that Ted was taken into care and looked after for a few days at a suitable centre in Inverness until he was sufficiently recovered to be transferred to our own little unit.

Gordon, under whose supervision the lad happened to fall, was a young man of breeding – previously an officer attached to a distinguished regiment of the line – with a distinctly phlegmatic disposition as became a young Englishman of his position. Gordon, therefore, was not inclined to lecture, harass or probe with excess zeal into Ted's affairs. Nobody set out to reason with the young man with the quasi-rational paternalism of the self-satisfied who are disturbed by forces beyond their comprehension; nobody thrust him into a 'therapeutic group' with its own stereotyped set of idioms, and nobody embarked on superficial programmes of 'occupational therapy' with its production of trumpery gewgaws, woollen rugs or bits of pottery, and nobody embarked upon the somewhat later versions of 'art therapy', 'music therapy' or any other of the rituals which conceal the need for patient support and opportune intervention, if only because we had neither the staff nor the need to engage upon fancy diversions from our privileged functions of observation and caring. It was also supremely important for Ted's welfare, as it turned out, that the major tranquillising drugs (which later contributed so notably to the naive belief in the pseudo-scientific cure of all behavioural problems) had not yet become available.

On the face of it, we did nothing in particular for young Ted; in fact, on reflection, we did a very good job indeed of doing nothing whatever beyond providing an agreeable environment, plenty of time and a suitably permissive regime.

Some weeks later, I came across Ted again, just as fortuitously as before. This time he was engaged upon a piece of work which took my attention not only because of its unusual nature, but very particularly because of the manner of Ted's commitment to it: he was securing half-sheets of illuminated vellum between layers of muslin, so that the text of the manuscript was clearly visible on both sides. Thus secured, each half-sheet was then framed between good margins of stout card, to make in all a permanent and portable display of the original.

Ted explained that the sheets he was working with had come from a medieval missal, and had at some stage been cut in half and packed together to form the binding for a book. He had the book at his side, and he was clearly familiar with this practice of putting discarded material to fresh use (presumably at the time of Edward VI, when it would suit the English Church both to destroy and conceal its unacceptable origins in Roman usage). It turned out that each mounted fragment had a definite market value which would handsomely reward its producer for his patient, sustained and diligent attention. There is something agreeably symbolic too in the supposition that Ted's work in restoring discarded and rejected material from the past may have been mirrored in his personal transformation from an apparent act of wilful self-destruction into the patient good-humoured and productive individual he had now become.

Nowadays, casual overdosage of tranquillising drugs in small doses is almost too common to have much general significance, but Ted's determination and his sustained assault on his own well-being were so much at odds with the tranquil and productive individual he had now become that the contrast took on an unaccountably striking character. Early psychoanalysts spoke of cure by *coup de foudre* (lightning stroke) – a term they soon abandoned, and with good reason; yet this young man's recovery had just such an effect on my own perception.

Illumination came about through Ted's remark that he had come across his bountiful old book at a local second-hand stall. Truly, fortune favours the prepared mind, yet there was something about this casual observation which I found in its own way as revealing as the unforced change in Ted's character.

At that time, the law placed very stringent conditions upon the admission of any individual to a psychiatric unit. It was then correspondingly all but unthinkable for anyone to be granted freedom of leave to proceed without let or hindrance, independently and unaccompanied, so far as the nearest town, where Ted must have wandered at will to browse among the second-hand bookshops. Such a daring step could only have been taken with the connivance of one man: a man of peculiar authority, comparable to that of a warrant-officer or a foreman, in this case the charge nurse of the unit. His name (and nothing else about him) was an odd one. Generations before, one of his ancestors had been Polish, and had bequeathed the name 'Pan' – simply, the Polish word for 'Mister'.

Harry Pan had an extraordinary range of qualities. He was reserved without being taciturn, realistic, consistent and decisive without ever indulging in any flamboyance or ostentation, and in addition he was as a private individual one of the most equable and agreeable people I have ever met. All these qualities must have contributed to the judgement and initiative which led him to confer upon Ted just the freedom he required to find his feet again and eventually make his own way forward. Diligent students of psychiatric history can find echoes of these qualities among the most outstanding pioneers of humane care: Harry Pan was the first of many whom I was to meet who embodied these qualities, and to evoke them, blundering through a thicket of words, is one of the most taxing tasks I have ever undertaken.

* * *

At all events, I had been far more fortunate in my first choice of jobs than I could have known, and in my first 12 months I had been transformed from a floundering student to being eminently employable. At the end of my contract with Professor Alexander, it had moreover become urgently necessary to secure another post with some haste. Postponing the uncertain prospects of a position with prospects of postgraduate training, I therefore tried my luck with an approach to Donald Mack, whom I had met when Sister (Surgical) had carried out her threat to 'get the psychiatrist'.

The patient in question was not in truth in any grave need of psychiatric care. He was an elderly lawyer whose neural network and circadian rhythms were getting a little into disarray, and whose surgical needs were not particularly urgent. His nephew had succeeded to the family business, and allowed him to potter about the office at night-time, no doubt having taken due precautions to prevent access to sensitive papers. Having once been the senior partner in a professional firm, the gentleman was not disposed to appreciate the hourly discipline of a surgical regime, and his absences in remote corners of the toilet suite during Alec's ward rounds had quickly stirred Sister into action. On his way down the ward, Dr Mack spot-diagnosed a couple of other people who were much more in need of his services, though also less likely to benefit from them. The upshot was that he and I had an agreeable conversation along professional lines, and arrangements were made for the (temporary) incarceration of the legal gentleman.

On the strength of this meeting, Donald Mack felt able to offer a suitable post without more ado, and shortly afterwards I set out again to trundle back across the moors to Ramscar.

2

Ramscar

Ramscar as an institution had nothing particularly notable about it at all, though its geography and its history were so singular that they compensated for what in the end turned out to be hardly more than a means of subsistence for my family. My modest worldly goods as a student were not finally redeemed from pawn until after I left there, but I relished its dramatic setting and the congenial warmth of my immediate colleagues.

Donald Mack, fortunately, was not an 'immediate colleague'. Variously known as 'Donald', plain 'Mac', or sometimes 'Big Mac' according to one's status and standing, he certainly appeared to see himself as the big man. He had acquired the position of Physician Superintendent after the advent of the National Health, having the irresistible combination of the right paper and the right connections.

His legal deputy, however, had been appointed by local government, and had not been required to conform with what later became the conventional appurtenances of authority. This made for a situation ripe with possibilities for political infighting, especially since a second consultant was in post who was a close soul mate of Donald's, and equipped with precisely the same qualifications, both formally and socially. This tangled skein of material could very nearly have been the stuff of which the hospital's traditions had been woven.

This ravel and cross-purpose was beautifully illustrated on the occasion of the hospital's half-century anniversary.

We had succeeded in unearthing the earliest records of the city fathers which related to the founding of the asylum (as it was then properly known). These records from the very start revealed a long-running comedy of errors. Having established an asylum committee and found a suitable site – which had as yet no means of access either by road or rail – it was decided that architects might submit proposals under a pseudonym by a given date. Six firms did so; two or three weeks before the closing date, a seventh firm sought leave to extend the date by a fortnight to allow it to put the finishing touches to its own proposals. The committee with all gravity of purpose acceded to this request, to the fury of the six contestants who had met their deadline. The committee had to rethink its decision, which in due course it affirmed. The heart-searching and the rancour which this involved are best left to the imagination. Thankfully when all was said and done, the latecomers were not successful in their application.

This was only the beginning. A railway line was duly constructed and work was set afoot. A typical débâcle occurred in the first summer of operations, when it was reported that the diggings for certain foundations were now ready, where a small but vital bridge was to give access to the kitchens. Permission was sought to proceed with building work, while the warm dry weather was favourable. The committee deliberated, and in its wisdom elected to appoint a subcommittee which might have the gratification not only of a trip to the country at the ratepayers' expense, but also the vicarious satisfaction of gloating over a very large piece of potential real estate. A subcommittee was duly appointed, then assembled and transported, and no doubt aired its knowledge, took its time, asked some Very Important Questions, and before evening fell, enjoyed its return trip to the familiar urban smoke whence it had come – and a month later submitted its report to the parent committee. Perhaps there was a summer vacation about that time, or possibly an exceptionally heavy agenda to delay the parent committee's compilation of a suitably weighty opinion; certainly, it was yet another full month before its agreement was in the hands of the builders. By then, of course, early autumn rains had swept down the hilly grounds, and the vital earthworks had collapsed under a natural assault from the torrent of a swift hill stream.

Once the vast institution was finally erected, there naturally had to be a Grand Opening. It should in fairness be said that the planners had achieved a truly splendid effect in material terms, in a spacious and dramatic setting, still impressive, adaptable and commodious two generations later.

Perhaps it was the size and grandeur of the setting which persuaded the authorities to encourage an authentic Earl to oversee the opening ceremonies.

This came to light during the anniversary celebrations. It fell to Donald to give the main address during the celebrations, and it has to be said that he did it remarkably well. Always a meticulous man, he had researched the period very carefully, and he held a large audience in the main hall completely spellbound for nearly an hour while he covered the main political and topical events of the day. He spoke well; he was always clearly audible, timed his comments splendidly and varied his tone at every turn to suit his material. The startling climax of his delivery came when he reached a detailed account of the opening ceremony itself.

Everybody had come by train along the special line with the sole exception of the Earl himself, who came in his horseless carriage – the only one to be both designed and made in the country. The noble lord proceeded to scandalise the entire gathering by declaring that the vast sums of money required for the erection of this large institution might have been put to better purpose by creating housing for his own farm-hands, rather than setting up a 'mausoleum for the living dead'. Having delivered himself of this shattering remark, he departed, as the press reported, 'in a cloud of dust and opprobrium'.

To judge from the memories of the nursing staff, it seemed that the hospital had run well enough during the period between the wars, when the superintendent conceived the idea (discovered in France in the eighteenth century, and briefly rediscovered after the Second World War) that physical work was beneficial for patients, giving them a sense of pride as well as helping them to sleep at night without the use of hypnotics; (effective hypnotics only became available in the twenties, and even then the night staff could have a hard time of it). This superintendent, Dr English, had left a reputation for diligent attentiveness to his charges' care; this was very often the case, though the larger urban centres were often run by men of very uncertain ability and idiosyncratic ideas, not to speak of a positively evil capacity for demoralising the staff. A superintendent's power was all but absolute and nearly always (there were notable exceptions) exercised despotically, subject in the days of accountability to local government authority to a certain sensitivity in matters of cost. (One superintendent told me with a wicked gleam in his eye that the way to secure a superintendency was to know where to buy beef at a penny per pound more cheaply than other candidates for the position.)

Dr English at any rate had the idea of levelling a large area of rocky ground, working with relays of men using wheelbarrows. Small wonder they slept well of nights.

Donald Mack's capacity for being meticulous extended to his sense of propriety. He never scrupled to avoid skulduggery if it served the hospital's interests as he saw them, but his care to maintain the appearances of rectitude was positively Calvinistic. This had the unfortunate effect that conjecture, or any genuine move toward innovation, was limited on the one hand to a display of textbook exotica or on the other to a slavish adherence to fashion or the appearance of progress.

Rather in keeping with this approach, he instituted weekly meetings at which we were all required to report any conditions of interest which had arisen during the previous week. One one occasion it fell to me to give an account of a man with an inconclusive set of symptoms among which, in passing, were minor complaints of abdominal colic. The man in question had been involved in dismantling motor-car batteries for recycling, and Donald was quick to pick this up.

'Ah, hm, well now, I wonder if he might be suffering from lead poisoning?'

The idea was not particularly plausible, nor was it presented as a remote possibility which should for completeness be followed up.

It fell to me to seek a laboratory report on the amount of lead in the sufferer's bloodstream, and there followed one of those exercises of indulgent courtesy which the experienced use in order to instruct the young and ignorant. It appeared that simple examination of the red blood cells under a microscope was at once simpler and more effective in deciding the diagnosis, though the laboratory would be happy to carry out the more demanding and less conclusive test if I wished. There was no laboratory evidence of lead poisoning.

Donald's general strategy meant that a junior member of staff who succeeded in some academic achievement would be rewarded with some slight, even nominal increase of responsibility. Much to his surprise, I had been successful at the first attempt in passing the preliminary part of a postgraduate diploma, and I was asked to undertake the assessment of a ward full of long-stay ('chronic') patients with a view to deciding which of them might benefit from 'rehabilitation'. No programme of rehabilitation as such existed, and although the hospital did have a large, enterprising and successful occupational therapy department (the best I have ever seen), it was full to capacity. I think it was expected that I would spend an afternoon with the charge nurse, and submit a neat list of sheep and goats within the next few days.

The grain of irritation which existed between us became evident two or three weeks later, when I was asked with an edge of tartness how I was progressing. I was complacent enough to be perhaps a fraction offhand; as a matter of fact, I was enjoying the exercise enormously.

There must have been at least 40 people on the ward, most of them in middle life or well past, and nearly all schizophrenic in one form or another, bearing in mind that 'if we wished, we could form almost as many groups as there were individuals'.[2] (My former colleague Trudy used to remark in her own laconic and forceful way that 'in psychiatry the only diagnosis is the patient's name'.) In any case, all my men showed what Henderson & Gillespie refer to simply as a 'general disintegration of all the mental functions',[3] resulting in an 'appearance of queerness and oddity, so striking to the ordinary observer'. The language was apt for its time, and our conversations were confined to the outlines of simple facts of what should have been common knowledge between us. The outcome astonished me. No one knew or cared very much about the Monarch, the Prime Minister, the date, his own age or how long he had been in Ramscar. Yet each of them was clear about his date of birth, emphatically clear about the precise day of his admission, and carried quite vivid memories of his wartime evacuation to the most remote hospital in the kingdom, in the far west reaches of the realm. One of them astonished me by recalling (correctly) that he had been at the battle of Jutland. One small paragraph of a standard text covers the situation completely, but the concrete demonstration that it is perfectly feasible to maintain even a restricted conversation on a rational basis with people apparently unable to care for themselves in the simplest way came to me as a profound shock.

I had begun to learn.

* * *

At the end of a year's service, Donald was able to offer promotion to a training grade with a salary somewhat higher than I could have had in the next 'service' level, with the proviso that I would not be entitled to the normal allowance of six months' leave for full-time postgraduate study. Circumstances left me with the uncomfortable obligation of submitting to the scarcely disguised threat that an application for a post with full training facilities would be unsuccessful. The immediate effect of this submission led eventually to a sense of insufferable restriction: the outcome in the longer term was to have completely unexpected benefits.

Meanwhile, the duties that I now had were simple enough, consisting of the day-to-day supervision of three or four long-stay villas, together with recording the condition and progress of patients on the admission unit. Both tasks were congenial, and demanded for the most part little more than following the guidelines of the textbook and of absorbing the collective wisdom of the nursing staff, often acquired over a generation of service.

The daily round of duties threw up some surprising rewards. I had an early success while talking to a man who had come in with a quite startling history of addiction to alcohol.

He was a tall, almost gangling man, except that he was lying quite still in bed, reclining on a mound of pillows, in a manner of repose. He remained quite still throughout, and his attitude was thoughtful, even reflective. He may have given his story many times before, though I think not.

At all events, he gave his history in a quite impeccable fashion. I had come to expect that addiction to alcohol was associated with evasiveness, over-dramatisation, and a certain florid display of false regrets and intentions of future reform, together with obvious physical signs of damage, but he showed none of these, except perhaps for a slightly greyish overall pallor.

He gave his account of himself in a measured, sober manner, fully and accurately. In a word, he was a good witness; had he been in court he might have been described as 'unshakeable'. I do not think I have ever met anyone else who could give such a steady and reasoned account of himself; if he had not rehearsed his story before others, it was likely that he had done a good deal of reflecting on his own account.

In fact, he had drunk his wife and family out of house and home, so that they had had to resort to living in a caravan. And then he had burned down the caravan. It was enough that he had done so; he recognised that further elaboration would be a detail out of proportion. (I guessed that he had probably fallen asleep with a lighted cigarette in his hand.)

It took him about half an hour to go through his story, steadily and without pause, apart from an occasional moment's rumination. For my part I remained silent: it seemed the only appropriate response. In the end he broke my silence.

'And you're only the second psychiatrist I've ever met that I could be doing with.' Then after another moment's break,

'The other one was Shaun Murphy.'

Now everyone in the region had heard of Shaun, if only because he had bought himself a new car on the strength of an anticipated promotion which failed to come about, but he was a senior trainee in the city itself, and it was entirely by chance that I bumped into him not long after at a case conference in the teaching centre.

I introduced myself and passed on our friend's implied compliment.

Shaun, it turned out, was a bold beefy Irish extrovert. 'Sure I remember the fellah fine', he responded simply. 'I called him a bloody fool.' Then he changed the subject.

This did not seem to me to be a comment which was completely at one with the spirit of the textbooks. Yet it had the ultimate accolade of the patient's sombre approval, and I began to wonder if there was some undefinable criterion at work which enables an individual to respond to something more than the spoken word. How ever could one believe otherwise? ('All meaning is socially constructed' – surely one of the very rare occasions when philosophers have betrayed their subject by approaching a common fact of life.)

I was soon to have another lesson in the virtues of undefinable communication. I never saw my alcoholic friend again, but before long I had occasion to go through the admission routine once more with a very different character (or so it seemed at the time). This was a man who had been admitted on the recommendation of the local court. He had been convicted on a charge of being drunk and disorderly, and the local press had reported that upon conviction, the accused had stood up in the dock and called down a blessing upon the head of the chairman of the court, following this with some vivid extempore prayer and an unaccompanied verse of some hymn.

This much I knew before we met. What I did not know was that he had the reputation of being a blind beggar. In fact, he was not blind ('visually handicapped' would in his case have been more accurate), and if he were indeed a beggar, he was not one who could have attracted the epithet of 'poor'. It is true that he spent his time either drinking or drunk, and either in prison (where he seemed quite happy) or in hospital, but he took some care to see that his circumstances suited his inclinations of the moment.

He had the singular name of Quintlan: Robert Quintlan, and he knew the ropes.

When I met him for the first time, the very weather mitigated against cordiality – it was winter-time, almost dark, and the remaining daylight practically obscured by total cloud. And I was hungry.

Bob sat hunched up in bed, his head between his knees, and quite oblivious to my approach, armed with stethoscope, ophthalmoscope, knee-jerk hammer and all the paraphernalia of the young physician. He showed no sign of paying any attention at all. I was angry and impatient, and spoke to him rather sharply in words of one syllable.

This galvanised him into action. He sat bolt upright, peering through his thick lenses, and with some force he retorted, 'Here, I'm a son of the Lord Jesus Christ the same as you are,' and more of the like.

For a moment I felt as it were the hot breath of the Medical Council's Disciplinary Committee down my neck – but from then on we were firm friends. Bob pursued a happy if somewhat feckless sort of life, and we met again on many occasions.

A colleague of mine once tried to cross swords with Bob when he turned up at the hospital demanding admission. My colleague – another Donald – was made of stern stuff, and sought to turn him away. Nobody got away lightly with denying Robert his fancy, and the said lad promptly took himself off and lay down in front of an ambulance in another part of the hospital grounds. The ambulance men prudently popped Bob aboard and obligingly ran him down to the admission ward. Donald was completely unrepentant, and asked the ambulance crew to drop Quintlan off at the local police station. As he had only just been released from prison, he was perhaps not unnaturally enraged by such high-handed behaviour, and took himself back to the city, where he presented himself before an alderman of some substance with whom he was in good favour. All this happened during one Sunday; the upshot of the affair was that on the Wednesday morning, the superintendent received a telephone call from the government's Central Board asking if it were indeed true that a homeless and handicapped man had been refused hospitality at Ramscar.

Long before tea, Robert had found his asylum again.

* * *

When my time at Ramscar came to an end, it did so quite suddenly, but the intervening years saw simultaneously two of those revolutions which hit psychiatry every 50 years or so.

One of these was evidenced by the introduction of effective tranquillisers, which brought their own consequences. The other was a renewal of interest in the practice of 'humane care'. This was demonstrated at Ramscar mainly by the use of pastel colours in place of the traditional three shades of dung on the walls, and by the introduction of unlocked doors. (The *Lancet* reprinted a collection of seminal papers under the title of *In the Mental Hospital*;[4] it went out of print very quickly, and appeared no more. It was far too important to attract any academic attention whatever.)

Historically, chronologically and from a methodological point of view, the use of drugs should take second place in this account, but for the sake of simplicity and brevity, it will be easier to describe experience with the 'pills-and-potions' approach (strictly speaking, the 'medical model') first of all.

A premonition of this occurred one autumn day when Donald Mack and I were standing together on the doorstep of the entrance to the main block of the hospital. A group of schizophrenic women were taking the air quietly on the large front lawn in the fading late sunshine in the company of their nurses. Donald jerked a thumb briskly in their general direction.

'When we find an answer to that lot,' he said, 'we can really get to work.'

It was not long before he could believe he was right.

My own first encounter with one of the new miracle drugs occurred almost incidentally after I had completed the daily round of a villa of patients. They had an interesting variety of conditions, but were mostly so stable and settled from one day to another that it was a matter of moments to go quickly through the living-room, dining-room and drawing-room before leaving again through the front door.

One morning however, as I reached the hall, I was asked to look at a relatively young man by the name of Tommy. For ten years, Tommy had been compliant and placid, but quite mute. Nobody on the staff had ever heard him speak, though it was perfectly clear that his capacity for understanding the spoken word was unimpaired. He had developed a habit of picking at the inner side of his right ankle, with the result that it bore a clean but gradually growing hole, where he had little by little removed the skin and underlying tissue. This was a simple problem, and I merely left instructions to cover it with a single layer of vaseline gauze and a light bandage, to allow any fluid to escape and the tissues to heal. As I turned to leave the hallway, I had an afterthought, and with all the casual arrogance of the young and ignorant, I called back a further instruction.

'While we're at it, you might as well give him a milligram of Reserpine twice a day.'

Now Tommy's elderly mother, a bent and impoverished lady aged before her time, had the habit of visiting her son every month, making the long and bumpy journey by bus each time to sit beside him and ask, 'How are you Tommy?' To which he invariably gave no response of any kind.

But ten days after we began to treat his sore, her visit fell due, and when she put her usual question, the nurses were thunderstruck to hear his instant reply, 'Got any fags?'

The staff were so excited by this totally unlooked-for response that they made a special point of reporting it on my next round. Reserpine is not now used, but the impact of its effect at its first trial was so dramatic that I have never forgotten it.

It took three or four years for tranquillising drugs and antidepressants to come into widespread use, but they gave dedicated followers of fashion the opportunity to discharge hundreds of patients in a very short time; and then, helped by the introduction of quite new classes of 'tranquillisers', to enlarge the scale of out-patient attendances quite dramatically, in an effort to help the very many people suffering from conditions not requiring the previously drastic step of admission. Fresh statutory provision also made it easier and less drastic to admit people for short periods, and to lessen any stigma which had previously attached to submission for psychiatric care.

The full consequences of these changes for the Western world remain to be seen, but Donald Mack and many like him had found some of the answers they were looking for.

The other revolution, the practice of humane care, was just as dramatic, but less predictable, depending on properties which are necessarily intangible: sensitivity, intuition, insight, poetry, spontaneity – of the dramatic, even. I saw this in action many times in the hands of particular individuals, and once at least (or so I believe) embodied in the traditions of an entire institution.

At Ramscar, two occasions in particular revealed how unexpectedly the human condition can respond to unforeseen changes.

The first of these involved a man whose appearance alone was striking and dramatic. He lived in the same villa as Tommy, who had responded so markedly to the use of Reserpine. His name was Andrew Collins, and he habitually stood just inside the entrance of the living-room, so that he was the first person to be seen on entering the ward. The grandson of a slave, he was a tall man, well over six feet, with a head of close-cropped curly grey hair. As a rule, he stood bolt upright at his full height with one ear close to a loud-speaker on the wall, and he wore through the fabric of his trouser pocket by means of beating against it continually with his fingers. As the only Negro in the hospital (the term 'black' was not then in use), his appearance was all the more distinctive.

But his appearance was not the only distinctive thing about him. He had the habit of moving only when he wished to do so, whether to go to bed, to dine, to bathe, or even to make way for others to do so. On one occasion, his static pose and his great height combined to bring about a swelling of his ankles which was so uncomfortable that he went to sit down in a comfortable armchair with his legs outstretched. I seized the opportunity to approach him with some very genuine respect, and asked if I might look at his swelling. On the instant, he advised me with some force that medical intervention would be an impertinence: he already knew more than enough about medicine. It was he indeed who instructed the professors of medicine at the university – yes, and the professors of surgery too. He himself took his instructions from God.

That was that. To treat him by force would have been ridiculous. Everybody knew him and respected his independence, and he co-operated perfectly well enough with ward routine so as not to require any coercion.

Consequently, as I entered the ward each morning, I passed the time of day briefly with Andrew Collins without breaking step and without expecting – or getting – any reply. I must have done this for a year or so almost until the time came for me to leave Ramscar.

'Nice weather again, Mr Collins.'

'Seasonable weather today, Mr Collins.'

'Bit cold today, Mr Collins.'

And so forth.

The surprise came shortly before I left the hospital and moved on.

It happened one summer morning that Collins was standing, unusually, near a small centre table bearing a pot plant – an aspidistra. A stray shaft of early sunlight caught the plant and showed it off to perfection. Collins called to me to go over and join him. His manner was firm and courteous. He neither raised his voice nor embellished his call with any invocation to the Deity or any reference to our relative social status, either conventional or in his own terms.

When I joined him, he indicated the main leaf of the plant.

'Look at that leaf,' he said. 'See how the veins are patterned so regularly. Look how the main vein runs up the centre of the leaf and divides into sections to feed the tissues: just look at the shine and the depth of colour on that surface...' and more of the like.

His conversation was rational, measured, even and coherent.

The change in his demeanour was so radical that I cross-questioned the staff carefully about any change in his routine management.

No, they said. Nothing. Except that the new matron had also spoken to him each day, just as I had.

Something had passed between us in those few moments which I do not fully understand. To call it simple human contact just begs the question. In the end, I believe that the currency of human exchange has some logic behind it which we cannot reach. Scientists, the high priests of the Western world today, like to conclude that 'clearly, further research is needed'. Except that, of course, it always will be.

Andy Collins was also concerned in the other revelation which occurred in the same ward. This involved also another man known simply and bluntly as 'the Dummy'.

The Dummy was a short, slender man with one outstanding peculiarity. He had a memory span so short as to be all but unbelievable. He had had some brain injury years before, the exact nature of which, for many reasons, I never enquired into. His conversation was clear and sensible, and his general movements to all intents and purposes completely unimpaired. His appearance, in all but stature, was entirely unremarkable. Yet he never knew his place at table and presumably was only able to maintain the appearance of a normal social life by virtue of being surrounded at all times by others who knew and respected local conventions. He stood in the same position all day and every day, not because he was schizophrenic or mentally handicapped ('had learning difficulties') in any of the usual ways – but simply because he could not sustain any plan of action for long enough to carry it out without clues from minute to minute to tell him what followed next.

I set out one day to carry out a rough trial of his disabilities. On entering the ward I went at once to the dining-room entrance, where the lad stood, and asked him if he had seen me before. Briskly he answered that he had certainly not. I asked if he would know me again if we met. He supposed that he would. So I went sharply round the drawing-room and returned to the boy's station no more than a minute or two later. Had he met me before? Emphatically not. (Oliver Sacks in *The Man Who Mistook His Wife For a Hat* has given a vivid account of a man with a similar affliction: varieties of memory loss exist according to the site of the physical damage.)

The agent of change in this instance was New Matron, a woman as despotically unpredictable as she was insensitive to the feelings and limitations of her staff. In her first year, she had decided that all charge nurses should spend Christmas Day on duty. Some complied. But in this case, Jim (most of the charges at Ramscar seem to have been called Jim) had for years run a steady ward without any trouble, and he saw no reason to deny himself his usual Christmas Day off on account of a matron's whim. What followed was rumoured to be a punitive act on her part.

On the Saturday following Christmas Day, Jim was taken aback to find a piano being wheeled into his ward, and before he had time to enquire any further, the wind was altogether taken out of his sails by a posse of a couple of dozen women – women! – from a neighbouring villa. A special tea had been provided for by previous (unannounced) arrangement with the catering staff . . . cakes, jellies, trifles, mince pies – and Jim discovered at last that his company were *nolens volens* to have a party.

When the nursing staff told me about it afterwards, they had been so flabbergasted that their accounts of the event were almost incoherent. But two incidents had impressed themselves upon everybody's memory.

To begin with, the statuesque and normally obstructive black man had got to his feet from the festive table and of his own volition launched upon a spontaneous and dignified speech of thanks to the management 'for this welcome if somewhat frugal repast'. And to cap all, the Dummy, no less, had taken a partner and accompanied her to a merry jig round the living-room floor.

This spontaneous outbreak of activity among people normally subjected to the forced, formal and artificial semblance of merriment inflicted upon them *en masse* by a hidebound hierarchy was a token of the liberation which was occurring here and there throughout the land. In the next five years, informal changes of this kind spread both in number and variety; not least among their benefits was a gradual loosening of restrictions in general hospitals as well.

One day, the history of these changes will need to be examined more carefully. It will take some diligence to do so with any justice to the conflicting moods of the time.

* * *

Ramscar had some curious virtues. After I left, I never returned to the hospital again, but it had provided a first substantial home for my family, and we returned to the district as often as we could to renew the personal contacts we had made there. These return visits were always rewarding, not only for the sake of strengthening old bonds, but also because the general locality had qualities of its own. That they were quite extraneous to the hospital is incidental. I have found them – even to read of them afterwards – intriguing and delightful.

The fact is that the institution lay in one of the smallest counties in the country, which still somehow managed to contain the ruins of a large royal palace, a tiny yet magical Stone Age burial ground, and a network of narrow winding country lanes which wove twisting up and down quite unpredictably through the rocky spine of the area, so that a leisurely exploration always left one feeling as though driving through a kind of wonderland where each destination came as a surprise to be discovered only on arrival.

Long after we had left, I read that the oldest known fossil reptile had been discovered in a quarry there, and with it a horde of giant fossil scorpions ranging from early aquatic forms through to more modern land-living varieties with suitably adapted gills. Scorpions three feet long, ancient fossils, ruins, burials and unknown destinations: more than enough for any disciple of Jung to ponder.

* * *

The end at Ramscar came quickly, but it came by a contorted route.

A new professor had arrived at the centre of affairs, and in the fulness of time he discovered that throughout the region there were people, like myself, who were being paid at the (slightly higher) rate for a postgraduate trainee, but employed on a service contract – namely for whole-time work – so that fees from postgraduate students were being lost to his department. Once discovered, this ploy was sorted out smartish at some very high level.

The first I knew of this was simply a change of title in small print at one end of a very long pay-slip. There was no detriment to my salary (which was meagre enough), but it did mean that there would be no further increments, and without any prospect of formal training, it meant that the game at Ramscar was for me no longer worth the candle.

I was by now sharing a small basement office with one of the most remarkable men I have ever met. He had retired from a post as a medical officer in one of the colonies which Britain still boasted of then, up-river as far as a boat could navigate. This meant that Bob had to cope single-handed with everything that a doctor could be expected to cope with – dermatology, every kind of surgery, midwifery, dentistry, everything. This was striking because Bob took his chance every so often to go into the city and sit at the feet of a Dr Tyler, a medical specialist who was known for his distinctive style of dress, but not, sadly, for very much else.

One morning Bob completely took the wind out of my sails by remarking in his own modest, softly spoken way that when he watched a man like Tyler at work – a man who had taught generations of medical students – he felt that his own life had been wasted. This was a view so completely at variance with my own that I was completely dumbfounded. Apart from anything else, Bob's life was remarkable in many other ways. He had had two families and survived a personal disaster of unthinkable proportions: he was simply content to have brought his children back to the city which had made him, and in the afternoons (which were usually slack) he spent his time quietly reading Aristotle for pleasure. He had perhaps more equanimity than any man I have ever known.

But Bob's temperament and his station in life were both very different from my own. I felt that I had, so to speak, come to the end of the branch line. I spent my time laboriously writing down premature speculations about Logic, Intelligence, Education, Life and who knows what. Our cosy little underground bunker was pleasant enough in its own way, yet even this became a kind of prison, since the Real World above us lay at the head of a stair which led to the admission ward (for us, literally admission to light, air, work and society), and at the head of that stair was a locked door which required a massive forged-metal master key to let us through. Each of us carried his own key, but at the end of three years it had become for me a monstrous symbol of tyranny that we had perforce to operate this cumbrous lump of stuff in order to gain access to a world where locks had been abolished – by fiat from the very authorities who could not so much as trouble to advise me of imminent radical changes in my circumstances.

3

Transition

Angry, and ill-disposed to pursue so unrewarding a quarry, I applied for the first three posts for which my credentials were suited that appeared in the current issue of the medical journal.

One position (in York) failed even to acknowledge my application: no shortage of promising local applicants there!

A second possible vacancy offered an interview within the week, and one grey wet autumn day I drove 60 miles along country roads to what seemed like a very distant and isolated institution. Isolated it certainly was: a great grey stone edifice perched high up on a steep hillside on the very edge of a large industrial conurbation. The man in charge was plainly overworked to the point of desperation; it showed in his face. I can recall standing talking with him affably enough outside his vast lonely establishment. I could secure the postgraduate training I needed at the university centre 20 miles away across country, and I was prepared to sacrifice my family's welfare up to a point in order to fill a position where I was needed and to acquire the formal paper which was a prerequisite to any real advancement. The position was mine if I wanted it, and I expressed my interest very positively, with one qualification. I had promised to visit another hospital at the weekend, and I felt duty bound to keep that appointment before making a final commitment.

Off then for another trip, this time for a hundred miles across country to the north. The day was bright, clear and sunlit. I chose the shortest route by the map: it was also the oldest and slowest. I arrived late, and at the wrong entrance to the hospital – outside the private wing. Directed to walk by a short cut, I abandoned my faithful old barouche and came across the superintendent taking his ease in the sunshine on the broad lawns at the front of the main block. Always quick on the uptake, he greeted me with the words, 'And what are you doing walking around the front of my hospital?'

He was equally quick to recognise the road I had taken (as indeed he should have been: he was familiar with every farm, every glen, every byway throughout the county). Escorting me then to his office, he put me at ease with all the skill of the true gentleman born and bred. With the same unobtrusive alacrity, he was gratified to learn of my previous experience, and continued in his own frankly rather artful way to make me feel relaxed.

'You have a family, doctor?'

Male chauvinist pride rose unbidden in my breast. 'Two sons, sir.' (The younger still in his carry-cot.)

'That's a good way to begin, doctor.'

And after a short pause as exquisitely timed as Alec Sutherland's had been in the darkling medical ward at Waterside, he observed, 'I have two sons and three daughters.'

Then, having trumped my ace without batting an eyelid, he rose to escort me round his hospital.

A short corridor led from the discreet suite of offices at the front of the hospital into the main building itself. The two were connected by a perfectly ordinary, undistinguished doorway, except that over the lintel there was a large marble plaque commemorating the original foundation of the institution.

It has to be explained at this point that I was wedded to the view – somewhat oversimple as it turns out – that the care of seriously disturbed people had begun with Pinel in Paris in 1792 and with the small group of wealthy Quakers in York in 1796. At the sight of this memorial I was therefore brought to an involuntary halt, considering that the date attributed to Hillside was 1781, almost ten years before the French Revolution.

I felt myself confronted with a testament from an era of prehistory, and had Dr Farquhar's breeding and composure not been so uniformly unflagging, I am sure I would have left him to walk on alone. As it was, he fell back and gave his approval to my astonished perusal before we continued our walk.

Dr Farquhar prudently confined our peregrinations for the most part to the spacious grounds of the asylum, pausing briefly in the small doctors' dining-room on the first floor, where we talked briefly about James Graham, first Marquess of Montrose, and admired a panoramic view over the coast and the broad strath where the gentle hours of northern sunshine served to ripen soft fruits for the nation's confectioners.

One building in particular caught my attention; a large, modern, unpretentious block in its own grounds, surrounded by a low wooden fence, it still contrived a sense of scale and elegance which suggested rather more than any local authority could have put its hand to. Once again I stopped involuntarily, struck by the contrast with the often rather squalid Victorian monstrosities which sprang up after 1845.

Puzzled, I turned to my guide and asked him which authority had supervised the hospital before the Health Service in 1948.

His composure momentarily shaken, he replied in a scandalised tone of voice, 'Oh, doctor, we were one of the seven Royals.'

I enquired no further, but little by little I began to appreciate something of what he meant to convey.

At all events, I returned home decided. I had to go to Hillside.

The telephone call which I had to make that evening was a sad one. Perhaps my potential employer of a few days earlier had already known what I would find in the lush wide spaces of the north, or perhaps desperation had become a way of life for him. In any case he was patient and understanding, and almost seemed to have anticipated my decision. His area was a rough one, and isolation can only have compounded his difficulties.

4

Hillside

Hillside was and is a real hospital. It has changed its name more than once, but its circumstances were so unusual (at any rate before contemporary methods took over) that it would be impossible to disguise or to conflate the place to any extent without doing grave violence to a very distinct and historical community. I like to believe that it was (and probably is) unique in its quality and nature; but on the face of it, Hillside – as it was – showed so many anomalies that a casual account, distorted by hindsight, could easily be read as a piece of ludicrous antiquity. That, it certainly was not. Beyond the vagaries of the time, and within the limits of its function, Hillside preserved qualities so remarkable that a warts-and-all sketch is the only way one can hope to begin to capture the essence of the place.

As in the rest of this account, the doctors' and patients' names and details have been altered to preserve confidentiality, but the community was real, and defies disguise.

I could believe that my reverence for Dr Farquhar's establishment was exaggerated, over-sentimental, or nostalgic. Yet of the junior doctors I heard of who worked there, to my certain knowledge all but two (at the most) went on to pursue psychiatry as a career to the very top. One became a professor at a British university, and all had heads harder than mine. Perhaps the place had failings, but there was still magic in the very air.

Everything about Hillside had a curious quality. It was

unheimlich, uncanny, and to look back at it in memory is as though to enter Barrie's magic forest where dreams come true and the 'real' world is left behind. The explanation is simple enough: Hillside had in truth inherited a rare tradition from the days of the plaque over the door, when 'humane reform' took shape here and there in the Western tradition. And it had apparently preserved its traditions unchanged for at least a hundred years.

To begin with, the structure and function of the medical staff were distinctly antiquated – one consultant, a deputy superintendent and three or four juniors, all of them to care for 800 patients. Dr Farquhar had presided over his staff and his charges for more than 20 years, and to tell the truth, although he did it very well, he was not a man for innovation. The day-to-day running of the hospital was therefore left to his juniors, while Andrew Farquhar did what he had to do, usually closeted mysteriously in his oak-panelled office or, in the afternoons, taking his ease in whatever manner claimed his attention – perhaps on the golf course, possibly engaging in private work, and often enough coming through to the little general office to engage his juniors in light conversation or to indulge in nostalgic reminiscence.

His deputy had a strange role somewhat outside the general running of the hospital. We saw him seldom, though we spoke of him often, and he played an odd part in the contorted politics of the place, as will appear.

The junior medical staff consisted of three or occasionally four young men. One of us, Bricknell, had qualified against his will at the instigation of his parents; quite possibly he had private means, since he had no ambitions at all towards securing promotion. He had been there for some years, and constituted a repository of hospital lore which was essential for any newcomer. He also had the ear of Dr Farquhar, since he knew the district and moved in much the same circles. He took the lead, so far as circumstances permitted, in arranging social occasions and supervising the fragile organisation of our duties.

These, as at Ramscar, were simple and agreeable. The hospital ran almost literally like clockwork. The medical day began at 9.0 a.m. – 'Not a minute before, doctor; not a minute after.' (Bricknell enlightened us one day that Dr Farquhar's dictum was strictly speaking in error, since it depended on the long-case clock in the superintendent's house, which began the week one minute fast by Greenwich Mean Time or British summer time, and ended the week one minute late).

At nine in the morning then, we assembled in the Female Admission Ward and proceeded in a leisurely way bed by bed round the ward. This was in no way an inquisitorial or even a narrowly informative affair. Dr Farquhar's instructions were sparing, frugal even, and mostly consisted of a delicately phrased hint that some action or another might have to be considered. His comments likewise operated mostly as delicate hints – an 'Oh, doctor!' or 'Do you think that's wise, doctor?' – and much of the time was taken up with sundry reminiscence or a fragment of local wisdom – 'She comes from Strathbogle farm, you know: that's on the Earl of So-and-so's estate.'

A short corridor led from Female Admission to Male Admission, and off this corridor lay a large empty marble hall. On one occasion we were delayed for some reason and stood together for a few moments, gazing around. Dr Farquhar glanced here and there, and after musing a little, dredging his memory, he remarked how in years gone by, any patient who needed surgery – for appendicitis, say – would have it done in that very room, which would be scrubbed, carbolised, and have a table installed, ready for a surgeon to be brought to the patient.

This morsel was accompanied by another throw-away line, which evidently tickled the old gentleman's fancy: he recalled how in times past it would happen on occasion that one or other of the kitchen maids, afflicted by toothache, would approach him diffidently and ask for relief. He was always able to oblige with an extraction, and the memory clearly gave him great pride and pleasure – 'I felt quite honoured, doctor.' Over the months, we heard this account more than once, and the doctor's modest glee in his paternal role never failed to communicate itself effectively.

After touring Male Admission, we would emerge by a side door to make our way to the main building, Dr Farquhar to his office and the rest of us to the pharmacy. Dr Williams, the deputy superintendent, supervised the ordering and issuing of medical supplies, which made for a separate saga of its own, but the little corps of juniors was responsible for making up bulk supplies of hypnotics (two varieties in quantities of a gallon each, made up once a fortnight with great delight in the weighing, balancing, mixing and stirring of ingredients); we also 'retailed' supplies to the wards. This had its own quirky twist, because Dr Williams invariably ordered large quantities of any new product offered to him by a representative from the big drug houses: consequently, we could ask him for a fresh supply of some tranquilliser, only to be told that there was a hundred pounds' worth of some other waiting to be used. This entailed a tour of the wards to alter the medicine cards throughout the hospital. No great harm ensued, since the pharmaceutical manufacturers were still busily engaged in tinkering with varieties of the same basic molecule, but the system gave rise to some mysterious complications for us to mull over as time went by.

These complications really unfolded as a rule about lunch-time, when Dr Williams could often be caught sight of hovering briefly between our own little office and the pharmacy door. Such conversations as we had with him would then be conducted briefly in terms of supply and demand (he was really quite a cheerful and friendly individual, but for reasons of his own he remained physically very evasive). Before lunch-time, a number of set pieces remained to be performed.

Pharmacy duties never took very long, and the next routine was another short, cheerful and nominal item which must surely have been in its last months even then. This was the censoring of outgoing mail, and was presumably covered by an Act of 1930 (which stated that communication with specified bodies was to be exempt from interruption). We initialled away discreetly, and if anything was in fact withheld from the post, it can only have been on grounds of complete unreadability. But we pursued our little ritual merrily enough and passed on to the next regular event of the day.

This involved a half-hour coffee-break with the assistant matrons. This was the only time when we regularly had an opportunity to engage any of the hospital staff in conversation, but we made an incongruous combination; one of the assistant matrons was a married woman of middle years who saw her position as simply a job of work. She was neither a dedicated nurse nor remotely an effervescent conversationist. A second assistant 'matron' doubled up as nurse tutor and captain of the hospital cricket team. He was too busy, too independent and too robustly cheerful to concern himself with the niceties of interprofessional relations. The deputy matron was capable of being both entertaining and informative, and under the influence of my wife's warmth of character she proved to be a quite exceptionally intelligent and enterprising person. She had made it her business to visit Russia, and took great delight in regaling us with accounts of the hospitality shown to her group. She herself had been able to visit an asylum in Leningrad, and another of her party, a Nonconformist minister, had been given the opportunity of occupying a pulpit in a Russian church and partaking in a religious service.

Maggie's personal life, however, remained quite strictly separate from her professional commitments. Wild speculations made her a single mother with connections abroad, but this might well have been a piece of Celtic fantasy deliberately manufactured in order to introduce a scintilla of interest into the general atmosphere of rural peace and calm.

Professionally, Maggie was a vigorous disciplinarian. If she set off round the hospital in the company of a doctor, she was quite capable of trying to take charge and lead the way, given half a chance; on one occasion I remarked to her on the wonderful condition of the patients' hair, which seemed to gleam and shine in the most lustrous way. She retorted briskly that so it should: every patient, every single patient, had her hair washed and combed scrupulously each week, or she, Mistress McFee, would know the reason why.

In her eyes, this was no more than good nursing care demanded. In mine, it seemed to symbolise an almost archetypal quality of dedicated patience and excellence which permeated the institution.

The fact is that junior doctors came and went in fairly short order. The hospital was known of for historical reasons, but it had no academic standing at all, and most of us moved on quickly to higher things, inspired, as I like to hope, by what we had seen. Our function in the scheme of things was not very clear – or rather, had we cared to be aware of it, our function was all too well-defined. We were disposable – competent enough because of our previous scrutiny by the good Dr Farquhar, but essentially there for purposes of routine care and maintenance. The place ran too smoothly, it was based on much too solid a foundation to be moved, moulded or shaped in any radical way by young birds of passage. As a consequence, we were thrown somewhat upon our own resources, and under Bricknell's sapiential authority we formed a kind of benevolent conspiracy, sharing fragments of gossip and wrinkles of know-how between ourselves from hour to hour and day to day.

After the vacant half-hour for coffee, one of us had to approach Dr Farquhar, ensconced in his office. This in itself entailed a tiny ritual which was passed on to each newcomer as occasion arose. Courtesy dictated a knock at the door, followed without delay by an enquiry as to his availability for the daily round. This was all very well, except that the stout panelled door had a 'slam lock', and no external handle. The dodge was to have a master key ready in one hand, insert it into the lock, knock with the other hand and open the door without more ado. If Dr Farquhar was snowed under by paperwork, we had to set off round the long-stay wards accompanied only by the senior of the duty nurses for the day. Normally, on the dot of half past ten, the chief would be free to join us – usually two juniors and an assistant matron, her presence more muted if the superintendent was with us.

In a sense this round was the big event of the day. Its pattern was invariable, but it took a couple of hours and was nearly always punctuated by the same landmarks: the lady in the private wing who would allow the door of her single room to be opened just sufficiently to report briefly upon her bowel motion of the previous day – 'a finger-length and a few small dots'; the corridor on the first floor of the private wing, with its panoramic view of the countryside; the rather heavy, stuffy Victorian furnishings in the same villa, and above all the last corridor in the main building.

This main building was symmetrical; men on the west wing, women on the east, each on two floors and along two of the limbs of an 'L'. After the first ward, on the ground floor along the front of the building, a degree of tedium and repetition set in; these wards were active and for them the day was already fairly well advanced. As we rounded the last corner on the ground floor, we were faced with the last long day-room at the end of which one final door lay between ourselves and the front entrance of the hospital. This too was all very well, except that a vigilant and articulate woman lay in wait for us, quietly knitting in a chair not far away. The moment that she heard a key enter the lock of the door, a stream of abuse was loosed about our ears.

'Criminals, villains, arch-murderers, I see you all...' and so forth.

Her language was the only violent thing about her. She let it rip with all the composure of a fireman directing a hose. We soon discovered that the object of her attention was really our superintendent, and her ill will was purely verbal. Just the same, her eruptions were so sudden and so beautifully timed that they could never be ignored.

This lady was one of a number of paranoid people scattered about the hospital. They made a fascinating body of individuals, likeable, intelligent, and normally meticulous in their appearance and their choice of words. Lesser degrees of paranoid characteristics sometimes show among citizens who may appear as useful members of society; to lawyers the become 'vexatious litigants'; journalists light upon them when they isolate themselves from society in lonely cottages and resist any attempt whatever to contact them, so that milkmen, postmen and other innocent callers are likely to be kept very strictly at a distance – sometimes with armed resistance.

What made the guardian of the gate so piquant in our case was that once through this last door in the main building, we emerged to go through the front door of the hospital itself out on to the broad lawns, the mature weeping willows and the broad vistas of the setting where I had first met Andrew Farquhar. From there we were able to follow our way round the rest of the institution: the small private wing, the large villa for elderly women, the little occupational department, through the laundry and the kitchen, past the spacious and immaculate farm buildings and back through reception. Rumour had it that an Act dating from the previous century required us to see each patient every day; in any case, the daily round took us up to within a few minutes of lunch-time, with one more mysterious ritual before we broke up and (as a rule) went our separate ways until the afternoon's duties.

The few minutes before lunch provided a hiatus within which Dr Williams might be found hovering uncertainly between the door of our office and the door of the pharmacy. This was the moment when he could be approached for medical supplies. The immediate response to such a request was apt to be unpredictable. With luck, he would simply dematerialise for a moment – or so it seemed to each of us who had occasion to approach him. It was not that he clearly turned on his heel and departed rapidly, rather an inexplicable case of now-you-see-him-now-you-don't.

This phenomenon gave rise to frequent discussion among our little corps. It was balanced by an equally mysterious phenomenon when, as it seemed, within moments he would materialise again, apparently without any noise or motion, carrying with him such items as we may have requested.

On one memorable occasion we asked for supplies of cotton wool, and instead had to make do with a fortnight's supply of rather rough brown unrefined material known as 'tow', perfectly suitable for mopping up sundry unsavoury liquids, though less agreeable for applying directly to the skin. There was no choice; the hospital had to put up with tow for a fortnight. The immediate explanation was simple. The lock on the door to the cupboard containing cotton wool had jammed, and nothing would do but that Dr Williams must unscrew the lock and put matters to right in person.

It was not our place to question the explanation, which as far as it went was after all perfectly reasonable, but it was months before the whole story leaked out and we discovered, to begin with, why it should take a fortnight to dismantle a lock, or why for that matter a carpenter could not have tackled the problem on the spot. This involved deep matters of church and state which went far beyond the immediate issue. Little by little the story unfolded.

The solution began one day when one of us announced delightedly that he had discovered where Dr Williams' cache was hidden.

'You know where the matron's office is? Well, there's a plain wooden door next to it, isn't there?' (Yes, that's right.) 'Well, that's a cupboard, and it's where he gets his stuff from.'

It was a good try, and partly right. Without knowing it, however, I had lit upon another piece of the solution a few weeks earlier.

This calls for some explanation, and imposes another metaphorical mulberry bush in our path.

It happened that our little communal office let into a large obscure cupboard; more of a small room than a cupboard, and lit only by a central electric light bulb. This dark and peculiar recess contained old bound volumes of case notes back to the time when the present hospital was built – over a century before – and the occasional need for access to these notes provided the only real reason for us to delve in there at all.

It happened also that this tiny chamber, this little cave, this repository of things past and things meant to be unknown, contained also a strange ancient tin trunk, as well as a minute clipping from a local paper.

This cutting assumed enormous importance for me, in the light of what was to follow. It was a simple account of the search for another site upon which to place the old hospital (which finally reopened in 1856). The mechanics of the search were as simple as the paper's brief report. Four members of the committee of management had taken a carriage and pair, and set out to explore the countryside for a suitable position. Four places were considered; one only was recommended. One of them was too low-lying and apt to be damp. Another was too exposed and open to the wind. A third had some other defect, and so the present site was chosen. (Its magnificence was one reason why Dr Farquhar had paused with me for a while at the small doctors' dining-room, that I might savour the rare prospect before me; that tale too has its sequel.)

This swift and effective enterprise came about for historical reasons. The institution served the public, but from its instigation until 1948 it continued to have a genuinely charitable basis. Details of hospital history gradually became known as Andrew Farquhar indulged his fancy when he dropped by in the afternoons to reminisce with his young followers. History was closely knit with practice; the nature of both was unfolded only gradually.

As for the old tin trunk, this contained nothing more than a sealed one-gallon jar of a concentrated sedative solution, a number of assorted bandages and some well-secured packets of magnesium sulphate and potassium bromide. Nothing, that is, except an invisible clue to the machinations of the amiable Dr Williams. This too was bound up with the history of the hospital, and came to light innocently enough in due course.

After lunch, the idiosyncratic nature of Hillside showed itself. Normal practice called for one junior to be on call for the rest of the day and the night following. Another would be 'second on call' and would remain available till the end of the afternoon. To be 'third on call' was a strictly nominal business which rarely called for observance.

Bricknell had established a *diktat* which asserted roundly that 'in the afternoon we play battleships'. This was an exaggeration. Sometimes there would be work to do – a new admission perhaps; possibly some minor accident or illness in the 'back wards' – and once a week a couple of us would slope off to the new university department of psychiatry 20 miles away. Then again, on alternate weeks there was always the possibility of an out-patient clinic, conducted in a fashion which only Hillside could have ordained.

Afternoons at the university department were always agreeable. The department strictly speaking occupied another (much smaller) of the Royal Hospitals, though the advent of the Health Service eventually gave it control over a large old asylum in adjacent grounds. The new professor at first had to make shift with what staff he could command, but he was a local man and quite unruffled by the enormity of the tasks which faced him.

We were always made welcome at the department on equal terms with the rest of the staff, and the same atmosphere of genial bonhomie existed as it had in the Observation Unit: quite diverse differences of opinion were tolerated with courtesy, and if a point of view were dismissed, it was always done so with good will. On one occasion I presented the case of a young woman who might, I thought, be suffering from an abnormal tangle of small blood vessels in the temporal lobe of her brain on one side. I was listened to attentively throughout; no one seemed to be greatly impressed by the possibility, but no one showed the kind of scorn which could be met with in the hurly-burly of practical management in the wards of a hospital. On another occasion, a learned young man set us a fine conundrum one afternoon, and when everyone (professor included) proved to be baffled, he produced his own proposal for all the world like a rabbit from a hat, and announced his intention of giving the patient a judicious dose of potassium the following day. The following week, distinctly crestfallen, he had to tell us that his treatment had had no visible effect; he had overlooked some esoteric peculiarity in the body's handling of the simple element. But nobody boxed clever for the sake of it, and there was a genuine commitment to the ultimate welfare of the people concerned.

Out-patient clinics were held on the loose-tight basis which seemed to rule everything. The sequence of events was invariable. Somebody would remember on a Thursday morning that it might be an out-patient day. Dr Farquhar would promise to ring up and find out (the clinics were held in small hospitals at some distance from Hillside itself). Sometimes there was no one to see, and so no clinic, no trip across the rolling countryside. We would turn out (and often did) for only one or two people. The Old Man would take us to the quiet little hospital in one or other of two little townships and leave us (with staggering aplomb) to see the patients and reach our own conclusions. The interviews were leisurely, as they should be, and after a suitable interval the chief would return, listen to our findings and go off to see the clients for himself. He was astonishingly quick about it, and would sum up a situation and form his own opinion in a minute or two. Sometimes he would disagree with us in his own quiet, decisive way. There was never the remotest hint of criticism or reproof. The decision was made and action would follow at Andrew Farquhar's behest. We ourselves took no further part in the proceedings at this stage and a leisurely run home invariably found us back in good time for tea.

Another major diversion was provided by the visit on alternate Tuesday mornings of a consultant physician, Dr Cleeve. Dr Cleeve had come from a senior position in the metropolis to take up a teaching post at the new medical school currently in the process of expansion down the road.

Bricknell reported in hushed tones that when he first came, Cleeve had taken them all aback by appearing in Harley Street gear – pinstripe trousers, wing collar, the lot. Evidently (it was reported) 'he soon learned to drop that', but he still cut an imposing figure.

In truth, his attendance at Hillside was an administrative ploy to allow the hospital to take on young doctors who were not yet fully registered with the Medical Council, but all of us enjoyed his visits – Cleeve included.

He was a tall, elegant man with all the right accomplishments. Quietly spoken and immensely dignified, he could still cut short a premature comment with a single glacial shaft of silence. He had two or three higher qualifications, played a mean hand of bridge, and in his day he had been captain of Rugby at a good public school. It goes without saying that he could move with ease at any level in society.

He would arrive in time for a little gentlemanly exchange of pleasantries with Andrew Farquhar while we for our part would pick out two or three people whose physical condition appeared to be problematical. The whole troop of us would then set off in an orderly manner to stroll ward by ward through the establishment. Once, and once only, there was an occasion for serious friction, but that arose much later and calls for a separate account. On one other occasion we had lit upon four people whom we felt called for a physician's expertise: Dr Cleeve was quietly obdurate.

'Enough is enough,' said he, and the fourth man had perforce to wait another fortnight for his expert opinion.

His duties completed, Dr Cleeve would retire gracefully to the chief's office, where the pair of them would take coffee together before resuming their normal routine. The encounter had an Olympian quality which graced our obscure fumbling with rare dignity.

* * *

One morning as we were leaving Male Admission, the staff nurse in charge caught my eye and quietly mentioned that he was having difficulty with a paranoid schizophrenic patient.

Since all my experience at Ramscar had been with patients from an urban setting, with nurses whose needs varied from requiring sympathetic personal on-the-spot support to immediate simple prescription by telephone, in a regime based upon the 'medical model' (a.k.a. the 'pills-and-potions' approach), my immediate response was to recommend a modest dose of morphia and hyoscine – an approach calculated to secure rapid sedation in nearly any situation.

Staff Nurse was flabbergasted. He took half a pace backwards and explained patiently and gently that morphia with hyoscine had not been used at Hillside for more than 20 years. He reflected for a moment and said, 'I'll just sit down and have a talk with him.'

That was it. No argument, nothing; just a simple quiet statement of fact.

I was bereft of speech. Nobody talks to a paranoid individual with a head of steam. In later years I have silenced paranoid outbursts either with a moment's genuine anger, or (once) by a few moments' attentive silence in a deeply pensive mood of dejection, but I have just as often made the mistake of trying to exchange pleasantries or to be sweetly reasonable with a grandiose and indignant individual in full flight. But the nurse was well satisfied to do his best, and I left him to it. (Next day, I discovered that he had spent an hour and a half in his efforts; they were successful.)

A similar situation arose again one morning as we rounded the corner to enter the last ward in the main block – the one guarded at its exit by Paranoid Lady Number One, the guardian of the gate, she of the vituperative abuse. On this occasion we were approached by a part-time assistant nurse, a small, quiet woman of great experience and obvious ability. She explained that she was having difficulty with a schizophrenic woman who was becoming unduly excited.

I responded at once with a recommendation of two other sedatives – milder, but effective in combination, and in common use at Ramscar. Nurse's reaction followed her colleague's. After a moment's reflection, she said that her patient was upset because her usual chair was not available: the painters had been in the ward, and the furniture had been moved. Nurse would put her chair back where it belonged, and have a little talk with the patient. Again it was plain that this plan was what would be adopted. Nurse was happy to try, and I was happy to let her. Years later a distinguished psychoanalyst with a commitment to research in the field of schizophrenia went into print with the discovery that schizophrenic people dislike change – change of staff, change of clothing, change of scene. Capable nurses had known it for years, and possibly for centuries.

This kind of situation cropped up again and again in different ways.

One night I was doing the rounds and making my way slowly and quietly down the main staircase when a peremptory voice demanded to know if I knew what I was doing.

'Can't you see that I am waiting? And take your hands out

of your pockets when you talk to me ...'

The speaker was a tall, gaunt woman in a long grey coat which effectively disguised her presence in the gloom of the large dark empty hallway. She was (yet another) paranoid woman, who wanted to go to bed. All the doors at Hillside were always locked. (They might almost as well not have been, since any patient who wished to go out simply stood by the appropriate door, and the first passer-by armed with a key would oblige without a word.)

I heard a lengthy account of this woman's story next day.

It turned out that her husband was a chronic drunkard who managed a small farm on a hilltop some five miles away across country. She herself left the hospital early each morning to go to clean and cook for her man, returning only when she was sure that he was safely home for the night, fed and comfortable. It appeared that one Christmas he had set out on a pub-crawl, and my ferocious acquaintance had taken it upon herself to follow him from each hostelry to the next, by taxi, remaining in the cab while he took his fill. Only when she had seen him safely home and tucked up for the night did she return to her own bed at Hillside.

Whatever the motives behind this strange and remarkable arrangement, I felt that it could only happen at Hillside.

Another night, towards midnight, I came upon an elderly lady in the private wing, lying quietly, fully clothed and wide awake, upon her bed. I approached the nurse in charge and remarked on the situation.

'Yes,' came the answer, 'it's quite all right. She's waiting for her son to arrive by aeroplane on the front lawn; he's taking her to Manchester.'

And there the matter rested. Anywhere else, I felt, Nurse would have earned a reprimand and possibly some reprisal. But not at Hillside.

Yet another night, this time in the large villa which had taken my attention when I first went to visit the hospital, I approached the nurse on duty as she was attending to someone in the vast dormitory. Asked if everything was in order, she replied that the only problem was with Agnes

McNab. Agnes, it seemed, obstinately refused to sleep under any conditions, 'unless,' said the nurse, 'I get on to the bed with her.' That stratagem was ruled out because, she said, 'then I go to sleep before she does.'

Nurse was not joking, though she allowed herself a wry smile.

I was so taken aback I asked her who had trained her, that she could conceive of so simple a human response which was at the same time so outrageously unorthodox.

'Oh, I don't know,' she said, and paused to reflect. Then she added, 'But Dr Short used to tell us "Ye must humour yer patients."'

I had asked the same question more than once, and invariably got the same reply, virtually word for word, and always with the same soft Scottish burr which lingers in the memory and defies transcription.

The point about Dr Short was that he had retired more than 20 years before, but his character so illuminated the hospital (and indeed the psychiatric practice of the time) that he demands a diversion to himself.

The oldest patient certainly remembered him. I went to speak to her once, early one winter evening. She was in her nineties, her sight and her memory failing, and at my approach she eased herself forward in her bed, straining eagerly in the half-light to see who I was. Hope sprang in her heart as she greeted me.

'Dr Short?'

Dr Short went round his hospital at least twice *every day* – except for ten days in the year when he took a holiday to go fishing. On those days he rang up his hospital each day to reassure himself as to its welfare.

Some of his nurses remembered him appearing at the bedside of an ailing patient, together with his juniors, in the early hours of the morning after the staff ball, in full evening dress.

Andrew Farquhar succeeded him some ten years or more before the hospital lost its independence, and quite soon after taking over, he felt it proper to make the short journey to Dr

Short's new house. Having done so, he was greeted abruptly with the words, 'What are ye doing here? Ye should be in yer hospital!'

Short was by no means unique. Another superintendent knew off by heart the name, birthday and date of admission of all his hundreds of patients. Another was able to pacify single-handed a man who was a middleweight boxing champion when four male nurses were powerless to act. A third, a legend in his own lifetime, was taking coffee with his juniors and expressed distress at seeing through the window a patient in an adjacent ward being manhandled by some nurses. Challenged by his young doctors to do any better himself, he put down his coffee without hesitation and did so. One gentle, generous man kept open door in his office to be accessible at any time to any person. Another pioneer became briefly known throughout the land for extending his services into the community. Many outstanding men left their mark up and down the country, mostly in the provinces. A few rebels made their mark in academic departments in London, pursuing their own individual ways with particular vigour. An oral tradition maintained that institutions in the capital were often run by half-competent eccentrics; it does seem likely that, here and there, a villainous and malicious man could rule over his staff and make their lives profoundly miserable. But the outstanding leaders had very special personal qualities, which defy specification except in abstract terms like 'dedication', 'vision' and 'enterprise'.

At all events, the ghostly figure of Dr Short helped to clarify what Hillside was about – it was about custodial care. In some hands, these later came to be terms of contemptuous abuse – in the hands, that is, of people who had not seen the emphasis placed on 'care', but rather on 'custody'.

The business of Hillside was, then, restricted, and this explained the extraordinary isolation, the almost nominal role of the medical staff in an organisation which appeared to function with such remarkable success. Dr Short's traditions were not, however, the whole story.

More of this came to light in the course of Andrew Farquhar's little tête-à-têtes in which from time to time he liked to indulge himself (they were invariably rewarding).

He chanced to remark that each year the old committee of management used to circularise the parishes it served, to the effect that the charge for its pauper lunatics for the coming 12 months would be so many pence per week. They knew, of course, that an extra penny per week would bring in £170 a year, and could calculate their needs accordingly.

'And of course, doctor, if they didn't like it, they were free to look elsewhere.'

(He relished the memory of their impotence and of the hospital's economic stranglehold. In one phrase he had explained the obvious quality of the architecture, the equipment and the estate. On a later occasion he mentioned that the salary of a Royal superintendent was twice that of one answerable to a local authority: this too had its roots in the genuinely charitable origins of the asylum.)

This also was not by any means the whole story. More of it came to light one day when he spoke of the monthly meetings of the committee. These were held in the town hall a few miles away, apparently being announced each time by the Provost's Beadle wielding a large hand-bell. Membership of the committee was held to be a considerable honour, but it carried a certain disadvantage. Many of the members were farmers, and therefore held to be men of substantial wealth, and so subject to the jibes of less well-endowed members of the community. As farmers do, they protested that their apparent prosperity was an illusion, and took no account of their capital outlay, the vagaries of the weather, the uncertainties of the market, the iniquity of government, and so forth.

The hospital authorities did their best to spare its committee members' blushes by writing down everything remotely feasible to its farm account, in a hopeless effort to conceal the inevitable profit which the farm in fact made. Evidence of the farm's prosperity was easy to see: the buildings were beautifully clean, spacious and well-maintained; a great variety of prize rosettes was displayed in the cowshed, and a fine herd of pedigree cattle had been kept until recent times.

Nevertheless, the accounts were published each year, and try as they would, the authorities could never conceal the success of their enterprise, much to the glee of a critical public and the discomfort of the committee men.

Dr Farquhar took an almost unholy glee in relating his anecdotes, but he had been brought up at a time when psychiatrists had plenty of time on their hands for speculation, and he dearly loved to mystify his audience with the same dry, almost laconic fashion which so became him.

'Of course, doctor, we used to have a poltergeist around here,' he mentioned almost casually. 'There was a young kitchen maid in the place at the time. When she left it disappeared.'

His comment called for no particular response; perhaps he liked to feel that he had sown a moment's disquiet in an impressionable mind.

One fragment he loved to recall; it was part of the lore which surrounded the hospital's loss of independent status with the advent of the National Health, and this narrative he always related in full, with all the detail he could muster, and a good deal of emphasis to boot.

It happened that when the time came for the old committee to give way before the National Health, it decided to go out with as much splendour as it could, and a final lavish banquet was prepared to mark the occasion. This was to take place in the large dining-room near the window where Andrew Farquhar and I had sat to admire the view. The chief would explain how the room was prepared, with the finest linen and silver, all under the eagle eye of Nellie, the head waitress. ('You know who I mean, doctor?' I certainly did: she was an immaculate figure who could stand completely immobile with that odd, observant stillness of one trained long years in 'service'.)

When Nellie was satisfied that everything whatever was exactly as it should be, she locked and double locked both doors to the dining-room – '*both* doors, doctor' – which was then ready for the grand function to follow.

When the doors were next unlocked, the large portrait of the first superintendent was found upon the floor. (It *was* a large portrait; prominently displayed in a central position, one could see it through the half-glazed walls which surrounded the room.)

The hospital engineer was asked to report; he found nothing amiss with the picture hooks, nor with the moulding from which they hung, nor yet with the cord which supported the picture.

'And what do you think of that, doctor? Nellie had locked the door – both doors – the engineer found nothing amiss, yet there was the picture!'

I believe the old chap himself accepted the impression that he conveyed. I am sure that if anyone had engaged in trickery, the deceit had never become public knowledge – A F was not the kind of man to keep such a thing secret – and at the time it would have been unthinkable to cross-question him. Yet 35 years later, a nasty cynical voice asks, *Who else had a key? Did anyone hear a fall? Could some young man have engaged in a subterfuge that he could not confess to?*

Personally, I like to believe the story as told. If it wasn't true, it deserves to be. And there was, after all, a poltergeist.

* * *

The advent of the Health Service had some repercussions which were not obvious. Some of these must have been lodged in Bricknell's capacious memory; others came to light only little by little in some mysterious way down the grapevine.

It transpired that not long after the National Health came into being, the new authorities prudently installed an accountant as hospital secretary. (This was because the perquisites of any physician superintendent were always lavish – they had to be, in order to secure the services of a man of any character – and those of a Royal superintendent doubly so.) A weighty part of the new secretary's remit was naturally to keep a beady eye on the superintendent's rights and privileges.

This little matter did not discomfit Andrew Farquhar in the least: he had a sharp eye of his own, and his position was secure. But the arrival of a trained accountant, answerable to a regional authority under a Secretary of State, meant that matters like stocktaking and expenditure were subject to altogether more rigorous scrutiny.

And that little matter bore quite directly upon the activities of Dr Williams. To begin with, a careful account of pharmacy stock was required at the year end. At first, this account passed muster without comment. But a year later, when the process was repeated, it was found that the hospital had mysteriously increased its stocks of pharmaceutical and medical supplies without any commensurate increase in expenditure. The alarm, the indignation, the turbulence which this gave rise to was not part of the oral tradition – at least not in any detail.

Dr Williams, of course, had felt no obligation either to keep or to render detailed accounts of his stewardship. Very likely he simply did not know, or could not be bothered to discover, precisely what he had in stock. What was known, and had passed into history, was that the secretary and his minions had mounted a *rastrellamento*, a mopping-up operation to unearth the facts for themselves. Apparently, they embarked upon a detailed search of the entire hospital, cupboard by cupboard and door by door. At one point two of them came upon a locked door which had no determinate function at all. One way or another they set about the grim process of revealing any secrets it held. How they did so without co-operation is not known, but when it yielded, it did so with a suddenness that took the inquisitors by surprise. It proved to be chock-a-block, stuffed full and overfull with rolls upon rolls of cotton wool, which showered down upon the ruthless public spirits intent upon their accountability.

Now at last we knew why there had been so much clandestine turmoil concerning the use of rough brown unrefined cotton waste all those weeks before. It was at last obvious that Williams was like a squirrel, with bits here, bits there, bits one knew not where, all over the hospital.

It was also known that the secretary was an elder of the Kirk, as was the engineer and one or two others, and it was darkly hinted that these few had formed an unholy alliance in the course of their ecclesiastical duties, when they could mull over in safety matters which would have been *ultra vires* at work. It was said that this conspiracy was extremely powerful and presented a serious threat to Dr Williams' position, yet the very odd fact of the matter was that we spoke of these things as though they took place in another world, and not one of us was even on nodding terms with anyone on the clerical or administrative staff.

About the time that this matter came to light, there began to be rumours – or suspicions of rumours even – that the superintendent might be beginning to contemplate the possibility of retirement. The only concrete evidence of this at first was an occasional habit he developed of pondering on the style and quality of the hospital's work as being perhaps unduly old-fashioned. His doubts were too deep-seated to be open to question, and to tell the truth the rapid changes occurring in mental hospital practice were giving rise to serious misgivings in younger and more far-sighted heads than Andrew Farquhar's. He gave no sign of knowing about anything going on in the world outside. The seven Royal superintendents had always inhabited a world of their own, and he may have maintained some contacts within that world, or conceivably somebody may have tactfully leaned on him.

At any rate, the next concrete indication was a request to copy the patients' histories out of the old bound volumes into new, modern loose-leaf files. (Previous generations had considered it dangerous for nurses to be allowed access to medical records.) The old bound volumes belonged, of course, in the strange cavern at the back of the doctors' office, and they make for a story of their own.

Before we had got very far with our transcribing, however, a couple of events took place which threw further light on Dr Farquhar's vision of his own role in the workings of the hospital.

Both events involved the great Dr Cleeve; the first was inconsequential, but it threatened to be interesting at the time both because of its medical interest and because of the triple conflict of interest which it threw into relief. It concerned a patient of Cleeve's who had been shown to have an uncommon and mysterious condition of the lung known as 'sarcoid'.

This woman was not responding to treatment, and Dr Cleeve claimed that he had realised that she needed the kind of long-term nursing care for which Hillside was perfectly suited. Most physicians would have taken a more cynical view, and simply have wanted to clear a bed for a more immediately rewarding individual, but I think that David Cleeve genuinely had a clearer perception of the woman's needs and of Hillside's resources.

Andrew Farquhar took one look at her, pronounced her to be depressed, and declared roundly that he would have her as right as rain within three weeks. Her condition came to my attention by accident as I was leafing through the new loose-leaf case-notes. The young man who admitted her had diligently followed the book and recorded that she was unaware of her whereabouts or of the year and of other facts of common knowledge – she was disoriented for time, place and person.

This meant one thing – that here was physical or chemical mischief at work within her brain. Without more ado, I arranged for a reading of her 'brain waves' (an electroencephalogram) – which was inconclusive. It involved, nevertheless, a journey of some 20 miles or more, and it provoked Andrew Farquhar into saying, 'Oh doctor, all this clever high technology.'

The next step was an investigation of the fluid bathing her brain and spine, by passing a long fine needle at the right point into the right space. Routine. But it drew from Dr Farquhar the further comment, 'Really, doctor, do you think it's kind, going and pushing needles into old ladies?'

But he knew that it was unexceptionable, and a laboratory report clearly showed a considerable excess of protein in the fluid. It was obvious that she had sarcoid disease involving the brain.

A quick search of the world literature revealed just six previously recorded cases.

We restored her treatment and she made a good recovery – for a time. David Cleeve allowed himself one wry comment – that in his own hands, she had improved when he withdrew the medication.

I asked him if we could publish a report. This time his response was more tart.

'You would need histological proof.' He meant visible proof at the hands of a surgeon – or a pathologist.

The fact is that it commonly falls to a psychiatrist to pursue a line of thought beyond the point at which the most learned physician is baffled. One cannot expect a physician to appreciate the fact, and even David Cleeve, who clearly enjoyed the excursions into our strange community, could hardly relish being put on the spot by a couple of very junior assistants.

The second incident was more serious. One of my sharp-eyed young colleagues had spotted a bed-fast patient lying quietly in a corner, looking very pale. A sample of blood was despatched post-haste (by the rural bus from the end of the lane) to the university. The man had less than a third of the red blood cells he should have had, but there was evidently more to it than that, because Dr Cleeve, for all his apparent composure, rang up after lunch the next day. He explained the need for urgent investigation and treatment and gave instructions for the chap to be transferred to his ward in the Royal Infirmary forthwith. In fact, the man had been a regular soldier on active service in Africa before the Second World War. He was an oddity in that he was a Yorkshireman, he was known to have had sandfly fever, and had been treated for syphilis of the brain. It says a good deal for Cleeve's dedication to his profession that he was prepared to act so swiftly on behalf of a bedridden man with no substantial prospects of effective cure.

I came across Andrew Farquhar in a corridor shortly afterwards, and explained the situation to him. He stood patiently at my side and listened attentively until I mentioned the prospective transfer at David Cleeve's instructions. Immediately, Dr Farquhar placed himself with the width of the corridor between us in confrontation.

'Doctor, you're not to send him. If the physicians and surgeons get their hands on one of my patients, they'll kill him. He's not to go.'

And he moved swiftly off to his office without bandying words any further.

I rang the Infirmary at once.

Cleeve was as lofty as only he knew how to be. 'Very well. If the hospital chooses to ignore my recommendations, it can dispense with my attentions as from this moment.'

Catastrophe. Useless to panic and broach the Old Man in his already defensive state of mind. Impasse, and prospects of disastrous hostility all round. Only one thing to do – appraise the situation.

And our patient saved the day for us. He died during the night.

There was a further twist. Hillside history still had a little to reveal.

We knew that the hospital had a splendid laboratory, small but beautifully equipped. Now and again we would let ourselves in, I think for the pure aesthetic pleasure of admiring the equipment. It had been substantially unused since the advent of the National Health, and was therefore a little disorderly and dusty – nothing disgraceful, just a little unkempt, and quite usable if we had had a mind to avail ourselves of it.

Now a post-mortem examination was required. A pathologist would travel from the city to carry it out. And arrangements had to be made for a table to be prepared, and the laboratory to be thoroughly cleaned and made orderly. So it was done, and a young lady arrived to do what was needful. I was away that day, but the following night I was on duty, and quite late that night I received a call from the distant city. An excited young woman identified herself as the pathologist and without more ado, so great was her excitement, launched upon an extended account of what she had found. The findings indicated one of only three conditions, all of them rare ... one occurring only in children, one in a limited area of the Near East. It was a particular rarity which she had clearly never seen or expected to see. So next day I printed the cause of death in block letters, not to confuse the local registrar. (It was actually Gaucher's disease, and as academic historians like to say, emphatically 'not my period'.)

That was almost the end of my experience at Hillside, and the importance of what I had seen is still not clear. I had, I am sure, been a witness to one very important facet of psychiatric history. Its origins probably date back to Arab culture of the ninth century in the Christian era. Its end may well have come about already, so far as Western traditions are concerned; but that of course is a different story.

One clue remained to be unearthed.

Shortly before I left Hillside, we embarked on the business of transcribing the old bound volumes of case-histories into a more modern loose-leaf format. It was a fascinating exercise.

The big black books dated back to 1845; the earliest must have been removed for safe keeping under lock and key, but the volumes from 1895 were certainly still available and still in use. Rosie, the old lady who would have preferred to see Dr Short in my place, had been admitted in that year.

The work had its difficulties, because most of the early entries obviously referred to people who had long since left, and we had to leaf backwards through the tomes to find the initial entries of the survivors. Unavoidably, a patient whose history ran beyond one page would find the next consecutive pages occupied by a number of later admissions, so that a single history of any length had to carry footnotes referring to the next (as well as the previous) page number carrying the same history. We were much too busy, therefore, to read all the early notes, but it was not long before a general picture began to emerge which suggested an outline of progress in the unthinkably distant days two generations before, with hardly any effective medication (though admittedly with the benefits of economic independence, superior architecture and rural amenities).

It seemed that the general management of a 'pauper lunatic' was to provide bed-rest for at least a week. The case-notes would contain a record (generally after three or four weeks) to the effect that the recently admitted patient was up and about on the ward. Much later (as a rule) there would be a record that the patient was engaged in regular work – possibly up to three or four months later. The past, of course, is a different country, and in those days 'work' could mean one or another of a great variety of things.

There exists, for instance, a remarkable autobiographical record of a woman who spent half of her very long life at another of the Royal Hospitals.[5] In her case, it would appear that there was a liberal regime for visitors, and numerous occasions for extended periods of leave. The author, patently a shrewd and lively observer, records on one occasion on returning from leave 'never was I so glad to return to the hospital': bearing in mind that she was a fisherman's widow living well before the end of the century, when social and economic circumstances were indescribably hard, it is perhaps not so surprising that she became glad ultimately to make her home at the hospital (where she finally died with her three surviving sons at her bedside). The point in this case is that she regularly worked outside the hospital in the nearby city itself, where she enjoyed lively and more agreeable social relationships with the ordinary workers than she was able to do in her native village, in which she had become an isolated social outcast because of her history of disturbed episodes of behaviour.

It has to be remembered too that a mental hospital (before the advent of 'tranquillising' drugs) was essentially a community: one hospital engineer remarked to me that many of his kind had been ships' engineers – 'After all, the asylum has everything that a ship has, apart from propulsion!' Consequently there was a wide variety of work available for both men and women, including laundry work, kitchen work, domestic service (for both staff and patients on the wards) and, above all, work on the farm and gardens.

At Hillside, the reception office was manned both by paid outside staff and by a patient (an amiable, gentle individual) with no more than a formal distinction made between them.

We could not have known it, but round the corner lay a second pharmaceutical revolution – the introduction of antidepressant drugs – which in an age intoxicated by high technology seemed at last to complete Donald Mack's blissful aspiration of 'finding an answer for this lot'. When that day dawned, it became fashionable to regard work as oppressive, irrelevant or uneconomic if it were merely valuable in its own right and not formulated from on high in order to serve some quasi-logical specifically therapeutic function. Hospital farms were to be forbidden by ministerial decree, and ongoing concerns which functioned in their own right with great satisfaction to all concerned had to be subject to nominal supervision by a time-consuming, ineffective and ill-assorted committee of 'experts' from a number of mutually uncomprehending disciplines.

All this was still in the future, and the resuscitation of ancient lore culled from the old bound volumes of early records threw another flood of light on the workings of the hospital.

For the 'bizarre kind of discipline' (as I had belittled psychiatry when talking to Professor David's wife) nowhere showed its character more clearly than at Hillside. While there certainly were many exceptional men in charge of the large asylums who knew all their patients by name and commanded general respect by the remarkable force of their understanding and example, they were still exceptional.

Andrew Farquhar was an amiable, intelligent, cultivated and thoughtful man, well spoken of after his departure as a thoroughly capable administrator, yet he was no innovator. He had inherited and nurtured a remarkable tradition, and like most men in his position, his function in all fairness was largely that of a figurehead, wily and perceptive in his response to political forces, but by no stretch of the imagination a man to be familiar with each of the hundreds of individuals in his charge. For the little bunch of youngsters who saw to the daily routine of the hospital, the situation was inescapably far worse. In sum, not one of the medical staff was closely familiar with more than a tiny proportion of the people in their care.

Yet Hillside had sustained a reputation for at least 150 years, and its influence was palpable for hundreds of miles across the country. Stature of this kind is not gained by a tradition of nursing care alone (the Quakers had achieved that very early on with the Retreat in York, but their foundation was and remained confined to the care of a few private paying patients), and it is not achieved by the existence of exceptional individuals exercising a personal influence through benevolent despotism; this effect can be undone in no time at all. A rural setting helps in many ways, not least because country people are familiar with natural rhythms, natural vagaries of fortune, and the need for far-sighted views and a willingness to exercise patience and an attitude of expectation. But above all, the rural background at Hillside fostered the provision of realistic working standards of a wide variety, all contributing to the common good of the community.

This I believe may have been the factor which held the hospital together, and which I had stumbled across during my own last days at Hillside, in the old notes which we had to rummage among in such a fortuitous way.

5

Betwixt and Between

Our guesses about Andrew Farquhar's departure were correct. He had as ever been very prudent, and prepared for his retirement well in advance. When the time came, I had already moved on to what I hoped would be higher things.

The first move came about as a matter of chance, following a lunch-time conversation during one of the quarterly meetings which the Association of Psychiatrists used to organise on the pretext of disseminating scholarship and erudition. They made, of course, for an excellent opportunity to enjoy a good lunch, to meet one's fellows and to enjoy a day off.

Somebody, recognising that I was not attached to one of the four or five centres of higher learning in the region, asked about my current appointment. I was happy to tell him, adding that I was not in fact engaged in any programme of formal training (postgraduate training was at that time still very much in a state of flux). This drew the lightning response that Dr Pearson across the table was eager to engage a middle-grade trainee.

The moment lodges in memory as one of those split seconds which affects a lifetime: every urge called upon me to declare my sublime contentment with the post I held. A rare moment of acquiescence stayed the tongue: within weeks I and my family had moved ourselves once again half the length of the country to acquire the magic piece of paper which might open the door to a position of apparent respectability and authority.

We moved on what seemed to be the darkest and wettest autumn day in living memory, and stayed for 18 months. They were among the most formative months ever. Ian Pearson was a young man who had taken office at a crucial time. He had inherited a modest 'bin', together with an ill-assorted bunch of medical staff who all occupied entrenched positions; local men with no more ambition than to earn an honest penny and bring up their families. The hospital, rather like the one I had been to look at before going to Hillside, lay on the edge of a large industrial city whose needs were met by a university department of psychiatry and by four or five vast institutions – as well as Bishopsgate.

Bishopsgate, to be sure, lay within the city boundaries, but by a very narrow margin. This meant that it enjoyed ready contact with teaching facilities and with colleagues at every level who could contribute a wide variety of expertise within a common framework of interest. Since I now enjoyed a contractual right to one full day each week in an organised programme of instruction, rubbing shoulders with a couple of paid-up psychoanalysts, an influential psychologist (they were still rare on the ground), a national authority on schizophrenia and some of the most expert practising hypnotists in the country, it might appear that this should have been a richly rewarding period. And so, in a formal and intellectual sense, it was. Not even Professor Alexander's unit could have encompassed such a range of abilities.

Two things, however, contributed to making the real rewards of Bishopsgate quite other than merely intellectual.

On the one hand, the community of interest which united the different departments of psychiatry, psychology, neurology and the like was as formal and academic as the material they had to offer. There was no common bond of loyalty between these disciplines comparable to that which Professor Alexander had created when he personally appointed the various staff of his own unit – the first of its kind in that particular university. Bishopsgate was part of a much larger region, and there was always a sense of personal choice as to where one's individual interests might lie, and a certain hint of potential asperity (most notable, oddly enough, among the psychoanalysts, whose credentials were perhaps less securely founded than the more physically rooted pretensions of medicine and psychology); there was a sense of awareness that different boundaries must be respected, that there were toes which were not to be trodden on, territories to be approached with sensitivity.

The working atmosphere of the hospital itself was quite different. The formal structure was much as at Hillside – one superintendent and four other doctors, with this difference, that each of us was perfectly capable of accepting responsibility for a number of wards on our own. We all met regularly, but we met as equals under the benevolent supervision of the then all-powerful superintendent. Each of us had some particular skill, and a particular style of working, well known and openly recognised by Ian Pearson.

We met each morning in Ian's office for a brief review of the previous day's legacy. Very soon after my appointment, Ian was delayed for some time, and I was left to the scrutiny of a couple of the others.

Where had I qualified? asked Gordon.

Well, in fact I had qualified at a rival centre with some claims to superior historical and political origins; a centre frankly given to adopting certain airs and graces. Not being a native of the place, I confessed my background, hastily disowning the stuffy and toffee-nosed atmosphere which it was widely claimed to have.

Jack Gibson, always shrewd of tongue and sparing of words, had caught my drift before I finished speaking, and retorted on the instant, 'Aye, *he's* frae there: aye, and he's toffee-nosed.'

So there was general recognition that we all had each other sized up. Any potential for serious friction between the four of us was, however, transformed by Ian's own personal qualities. He had a capacity of perceptiveness combined with a quality of candour which made him superbly well-equipped for his post. The open recognition of our virtues and failings made for a frankness in our dealings with each other which was never tinged with any air of conspiracy. Even more, Ian's authority and his personal qualities of benevolent supervision extended to all members of his staff, so that all of us were free to engage in reasonably jovial personal exchanges without the acrimony which normally pervades a large institution.

Nursing staff, clerical staff (unusually) and artisans were all free to communicate on a personal level, with a curious effect of creating an overall air of harmony and goodwill which never descended to the level of becoming an elaborate comedy of manners, and never lost touch with a commitment to providing the best service we could in the interests of the common good.

The second feature of life at Bishopsgate which made for frankly healthy and satisfying conditions of work had its origins in historical and geographical circumstance. Antidepressant drugs and the 'minor tranquillisers' (Librium, Valium and the rest) were not yet available, and the 'major tranquillisers', the 'antipsychotic' derivatives of phenothiazine, had not yet achieved such widespread use as they later acquired.

Once people became more thoroughly convinced that Donald Mack's plaintive aspiration of 'an answer for these people' – those other people – had been achieved, boundaries seemed to have been broken, floodgates opened, and a torrent of hitherto undreamed-of problems released, with unimaginably far-reaching consequences.

Bishopsgate had not yet been swamped (as it was ultimately to be swept away) by this inundation. In addition, its somewhat remote position meant that the more straightforward problems could be sorted out at one of the units nearer to the city centre. Only the few with particularly adverse social circumstances or who seemed likely to present long-term difficulties were sent out to our rather isolated establishment. And only Gordon and Ian himself travelled in to one of the large general hospitals to see a handful of out-patients. Gordon had steeped himself in Pavlovian lore, and would trot out his own line of patter for all the world like a fundamentalist adherent relishing his verses of scripture, long before the psychologists developed and refined their own behavioural therapies.

Consequently the rest of us had a relatively easy life. Ian's oversight represented neither a grudging concession to tradition (as might possibly have been said of Hillside) nor was it driven by fashion and by intellectual aspiration (as it seemed to me that Ramscar had been). He was a thoughtful, even contemplative man, with a flair for administration which was as vigorous, effective and skilful as it was patient and unostentatious.

The relaxed but attentive atmosphere which resulted meant that every patient could be approached, at least in principle, in a conversational way, with far more satisfying results than the stilted and formal attack dictated by slavish adherence to the textbooks. As in the early days of my spell at Ramscar, it became possible to enjoy a far richer relationship with schizophrenic patients (mostly) than was usually accepted as feasible.

Three people in particular linger in the memory. I had been entrusted with supervision of the admission ward for women, and two of the people whom I remember especially had come into hospital for the first time; possibly this accounts for the ease with which it was possible to make a relationship with them, since they could not have been exposed to the conditions making for 'institutional neurosis'. (This condition was described with great éclat a couple of years later – just in time for its disappearance.)

One of the three was a young woman who was controlled by an invisible boyfriend. Her symptoms were quite startling; unusual in their nature and in the clarity with which she displayed them. Any question was met with an attentive silence.

'How old are you, Miss Roberts?'

(Attentive pause.) 'He says I've to tell you I'm eighteen.'

'Where were you born, Miss Roberts?'

(Another pause, head cocked to one side, listening.) 'He says I've to tell you it was in Paisley.'

And so the conversation went on. It was all a little bizarre, as indeed one had to expect, but it was also quite unlike the garbled word-salad which one could commonly encounter without preamble from some total stranger in one of the corridors between the long-stay wards.

The second of the three people who lodge especially in the memory was a slim, quiet, well-dressed woman in her fifties. Her symptoms escape me now; probably she had a paranoid form of disorder, but the abiding memory is of a well-spoken, quiet and thoroughly likeable woman. I do remember that she had been born on a small island among the Inner Hebrides (which no doubt accounted for the soft and melodious quality of her voice). Just possibly, in that one brief encounter, as with Andrew Collins at Ramscar, something had passed between us which is not entirely comprehensible.

But the third encounter which lodges in memory does so for all the world like a bone in the throat: it was entirely comprehensible, and no less illuminating for that.

The third meeting was under different circumstances, unplanned, unforeseen, unheralded. It was on a Sunday morning, in foreign territory, during what should have been a routine round of the hospital as the duty man for the weekend, and I was approached in the precipitate way which (some) schizophrenics have, by a man, a stranger to me, who quite clearly and with some urgency expressed a wish to go home – and that forthwith.

I was caught unawares, and resorted to a piece of devious rationalisation which did not for a moment deceive my inquisitor: I had the brazen effrontery to suggest to him with the loftiest aplomb that it might be a matter of courtesy to approach his regular medical attendant on the following day. Just as Jack Gibson had done on a previous occasion, he caught my drift before my pretty speech was finished, and on the instant he turned away, muttering and hallucinating incontinently, 'Do ye hear that, ye buggers...?'.

None of these encounters added essentially to the experiences I had had at Ramscar. The really interesting feature of the situation was the light it threw upon the nature of knowledge – or better, upon the nature of knowing. If the practice of psychiatry taught me any one lesson more than another, it was that the unexpected, the unaccountable, is always likely to irrupt upon the scene. This is perhaps a little beside the point in the context of understanding schizophrenic patients, but it does show itself in two ways – first through the unforced attempt to engage in some sort of dialogue in a more basic way than words can convey, and second, in finding more to a situation than one has attributed to it.

To put this more plainly (and remembering that what applies to schizophrenic types of disorder may also apply to lesser degrees of disturbance as well), we can consider, first, that the formal textbooks are quite clear about the quality of a patient's memory and the retention of 'general intellectual faculties', and second, that any nurse worthy of her salt will 'know' not only 'what makes a man tick', but also that her schizophrenic patient retains some at least of the quite complex skills which he possessed before his general social capacities disintegrated. Some (exceptional) psychiatrists did so too, yet the surprising fact of the matter is that the general rule was to assume that the schizophrenic patient was something quite other, quite beyond any capacity for making or responding to any human relationship. I had perhaps made this mistake myself when taken unawares on strange ground of a Sunday morning. On reflection, I am inclined to believe that the mistake is more basic than that of dismissing severe disturbance as being quite beyond comprehension and not deserving of effort: it is, I suspect, part and parcel of the failure to recognise and respond to what people are about. It is this difficulty of empathy, I would suggest, which makes the idea of an Unconscious so intractable and so uncomfortable, so unsettling – and not least for those who make it their profession (vocation?) to investigate its ways.

Be that as it may, I certainly came across one experienced and senior psychiatrist (admittedly labouring under early training in the metropolis) who refused point-blank to accept the idea that a schizophrenic patient of his could have reacted to a change of circumstance (as he undoubtedly had). He was by no means exceptional: a chief examiner for the College of Psychiatrists has recorded how at this period in provincial English hospitals 'it would have been unusual as a visitor to have a coherent conversation with a patient; yet whenever I tried to do so, *I was always a bit surprised by the amount of sanity which existed in even the most dishevelled or bizarre person.*'[6]

I think this problem, in principle, lies at the heart of psychiatric history: its literature belongs with the writings of the anti-psychiatrists (that is, with those who have practical experience in the field; certainly not with French intellectuals or English-speaking sociologists sporting fine reputations and rich pickings from furious displays of radical chic within the safety of their ivory towers).

For young trainees, it was perhaps natural that we should have been intrigued by examples of complex skills and of sensitive reactions existing among 'even the most dishevelled and bizarre persons'. On the same ward (at Ramscar) which housed Andrew Collins and the Dummy, for example, the nursing staff took pride in bringing to my attention a man with a 'hebephrenic' variety of schizophrenic affliction. He usually spent his time pacing around the ward in a frenzied kind of way, muttering and chattering to himself in a quite incomprehensible fashion. He had been a motor mechanic, and the staff maintained that he could identify any car which passed the windows, along the main drive through the hospital, by make, model and year, and invited me to put him to the test. He was called across, and came at once. There and then, on the spot, he verified and demonstrated his ability, and prompted by the staff, he went on to expound a trick of the trade by means of which a car could be decarbonised at the knock-down price of one pound sterling for each cylinder. (The dodge was to remove sparking plugs, pipe in oxygen from a large cylinder to each one of the car's, and drop in a lighted match. His description of the 'whoosh' which followed was beautifully graphic, and his delight in the trickery quite unfeigned.)

Again, a learned medical friend of mine at another hospital (another 'Royal') described with some astonishment how a schizophrenic patient was placed in the institution's cricket team entirely on his merits. This man would apparently be posted in the outfield, where he would hallucinate furiously, to all appearances quite unaware of the broad wide world about him. Until, that is, a ball should appear in his direction, when his skill at interception was displayed to fine advantage.

Finally, the staff at Hillside had a sad little history of their own to relate.

Hillside too had its cricket team, staff and patients alike, again chosen on the sole criterion of merit. One particular match each year had long been a needle match: the opposing team came from another hospital. As I remember, that hospital had been evacuated from a major urban centre during the war, and fierce rivalry had been sustained ever afterwards, even across a hundred miles and more of intervening countryside.

The regular opening batsman was epileptic (the term is descriptive, and not diagnostic; nor had the sophisticated pharmaceuticals of today been introduced at the time). But sadly, he had in some way been deemed to have been misbehaving in the days running up to the great match itself, and it was held to be fit and proper that he be deprived of his privilege and not allowed to attend the game. So great was his fury that he embarked upon a series of convulsions from which he never recovered. A benevolent psychotherapist assures me blandly that convulsions upon the couch are, if not a matter of course, at any rate no cause for alarm. For my part, the reciprocal influences of mind and body still offer unfathomable scope for observation and attention.

* * *

Bishopsgate was so much a watershed in terms of experience, and of psychiatric history too, that it makes a suitable point to reflect on the one episode at Hillside which could convince me that there really were 'bad old days'. Hillside, perhaps because it was a 'public subscription asylum'[7] seems to have avoided the cramped 'airing-courts', the segregation *en bloc* of acutely suicidal patients, and most of the other horrors of English municipal institutions; but it had retained one feature which only went out of fashion as a general rule after the wholesale adoption of major tranquillising drugs: this was the use of a single common dining-room for meals. (Christian Watt, an astute observer, records her horror of this practice at another Royal asylum.)[8]

I had become aware of this quite by accident one day on leaving the doctors' office to go for my own lunch a little earlier than usual. I emerged, all unwitting, into the main corridor of the hospital in order to cross it on the way out. The staff very rarely used this route, which was quite a modest and unobtrusive construction (unlike the vast, forbidding thoroughfares so characteristic of its large English counterparts), and to my horror I found that the length of a few paces which should have taken me out to liberty was barred by a packed mass of hundreds of male residents shuffling *en masse* with a kind of *marche à petits pas*, their faces grey and expressionless, arms bent at the elbow and voices stilled, the very picture that was to be depicted as 'institutional neurosis'.

The long memories of Dr Farquhar and of his nursing staff, it is true, did throw up isolated anecdotes of untoward events: a gruesome account of a man who succeeded in achieving his own castration; a bizarre suicide by drowning in inches of water, an isolated act of what sounded like quite unnecessary cruelty by a doctor (30 years in the past), but nothing like the routine ghastliness which we are asked to believe as being the daily practice of asylum care. The image of that mass feeding-time was the only evidence I had seen in five years of experience which suggested any degradation in the standards of humane care which had been typical of best practice for one and a half centuries.

At a later date, and in a quite different hospital, I heard accounts which led one to suppose that elsewhere matters were rather different.

One especially shrewd and experienced charge nurse described with horror his early days as a young man between the wars, driven by economic necessity to accept a position on the staff of his local institution. It had then been the habit for staff and patients alike to spend their daylight hours out of doors in all weathers in an 'airing-court', bounded by tall, stout, iron railings. Come rain, come snow, inmates (I was told) circulated all day within the confines of this court, while the staff remained posted (so it was said) each at his own position according to his rank and experience, day in, day out. It had been for all the world like a realisation of Van Gogh's prison with an inflated population. My friend could make the flesh creep with his account of the distant past – though he did have a singular gift for dramatisation.

* * *

One event at Bishopsgate stands apart from all the rest. For a long time, I felt that it had represented a lack of feeling on my own part. Half a lifetime later, with the evidence of similar situations and more mature conjecture, I am not so sure.

What happened was simple in itself, yet so striking in its context, so unexpected that it made for an epiphany which was not repeated for many years to come.

One afternoon, towards teatime, I was informed that we were to have an emergency admission, a young woman to be detained under compulsion ('certified'). She had been detained for a spell at Bishopsgate before, and was 'subnormal,' epileptic and of Irish extraction. If I could have dealt with the situation expeditiously, as a quick, routine procedure, this disruption of the normal, even tenor of life would not have been in the least disturbing; but when I reached the admission ward, the nurses told me as a matter of some urgency that the young woman would like to have a word with me before the admission procedure went any further. I was distinctly nettled, to say the least, by what I saw as an imperious assault on the hospital's authority, and responded somewhat sharply to the nurse's request. I would see her, I said, when I was ready.

And so I did. I found her previous notes, assembled the necessary forms and made myself comfortable in the ward office, taking plenty of time, and finally assumed a suitable couch-side manner.

The girl's story was unusual. Her mother had died a couple of days before, and was to be buried the next day. The body lay in its coffin at the family home, with large candles burning nearby. The only other member of the family had had to go out for a loaf of bread and some milk, and as she left the house, the draught from the doorway had momentarily blown the curtains at the window into the flame of one of the candles. A curtain caught fire, and very quickly there was a substantial conflagration, enough to cause some charring of the coffin.

The lassie had gone out into the street, and there was some general hurly-burly before matters were brought under control, but in the process some quick-thinking, right-minded citizen had disposed of the distraught youngster by invoking the authorities and removing her to the distant security of the asylum.

What was (and remains) astonishing is the manner with which this history was revealed. This girl, who had so recently been in the middle of an unimaginably horrifying predicament, and faced with her mother's burial on the following day, gave her story with absolute dignity and composure. She put it to me that she would like to return home in time for the ceremony, and she did so with considerably less anxiety than the nurses had shown when I entered the ward. She told me the facts and posed her request, without for a moment presuming upon the outcome. It was now I who needed help, and I sought it from Dr Pearson.

He heard me out, advised me that the hospital was not compelled to detain any patient, and explained that he was unfortunately too heavily engaged at the moment to be able to give the matter his personal attention; I must make up my own mind. I decided to take a break, and went for tea until I had had time for reflection. Ian rang me while I was still deliberating. He had made time to see her for himself; his opinion was the same as mine, and the young woman was home before nightfall.

The incident stands out with a force which I find hard to explain. An almost identical situation arose many years later (see Chapter 9); the memory of both occasions still brings my thinking to a halt.

6

Catastrophe

I had been far luckier than I knew in my first choices of post. But at Bishopsgate I had collected the paper I needed in order to look for promotion, and with headlong impetuosity I applied for the first likely position which offered substantially better prospects.

Brightways was half the kingdom away, but I had visited the area once 20 years before, and I knew the neighbouring counties. The hospital was, however, on the very edge of its administrative region, and so undistinguished that a colleague who joined the staff at a later date was told quite firmly that it did not exist!

In fact, the introduction of the major tranquillising drugs had coincided with the retirement of the last of the old despotic, omnipotent superintendents, so that the place had enjoyed a whirlwind transformation both physically and ideologically. I managed to catch it wrong-footed, as it was changing into the very model of a modern mental hospital: that is to say, at the beginning of a long turbulent process leading to its demolition.

The subsequent history of the place mirrored in microcosm the broad history of Western psychiatry in general, but it was hideously distorted by the personal qualities of the senior medical staff, who all unwitting paved the way for the political and administrative changes reflecting the spirit of the age.

For instance, George, the current superintendent, had barely had time to settle in to his new position; and to make matters worse, his deputy was a man of diametrically opposed temperament and views. (It seems to have been standard practice to engage superintendents and deputies who never communicated if they could help it: in earlier days at another provincial hospital, a chief and his deputy had descended to fisticuffs because both of them wanted the use of the only available syringe on a ward, and at another particularly remote institution, the only junior member of medical staff resigned his post rather than continue to be the only intermediary between his seniors.)

George was a chronically anxious and obsessional individual, not to say dishonest and doubtfully competent (over the years, he grew to be a gentle and well-liked old man, but his virtues lay dormant for a good many years before changing circumstances left him feeling secure enough to reveal them). He had an essentially provincial view of life, and his prejudices were very deeply rooted in the metropolitan traditions of his time – that is to say, in a thoroughly physical and sceptical approach to his work, apparently devoid of any capacity for either intuition or empathy.

He himself attributed his devotion to physical and chemical methods to his admittedly appalling experiences in backward and old-fashioned establishments. This was, however, by no means the whole story, because British psychiatry of the day was very heavily influenced (almost dominated) by a figure who had been equally appalled by the misery to which his patients were reduced, and who had shown a quite extraordinary vigour in using any available physical or chemical means in order to relieve their distress. The remarkable thing about this thoroughly outstanding character was that he could achieve results which his own followers could not duplicate even by the use of his own methods. On one occasion, he was matched in a brief and mannerly broadcast debate against an eminent medical psychoanalyst (who did his utmost to deny any use of drugs whatever in his own specialised unit). In this debate it was the psychoanalyst who in the event succeeded in having the last word.

'I can only say, doctor, that if you get the results which you say that you do, then you must be a better psychiatrist than you make yourself out to be.'

The analyst was right, if not entirely in the sense in which he intended his words. By a quirk of fate I was to meet up with his pre-eminent protagonist in another broadcasting studio many years later. My own sympathies were broadly speaking much more inclined to the analytic, psychological approach to life; I was therefore astonished to find that my very distinguished companion, whose views, on paper at least, were so divergent from my own, turned out to be an entirely charming and affable man. Brightways was completely unknown to him, and I had to describe its geography in some detail before he was satisfied of its existence, but the warmth and candour of his personality enfolded one almost tangibly. This quality of being able to communicate his feeling was, I am sure, what marked him out as a quite exceptional worker.

George, however, driven by the same conscious motives, remained a cold, frightened man, quivering with horror at every managerial or administrative whim, so frightened by the potential incapacity of his long-stay patients that he did all he could to deny their existence. His dread of them was so nearly absolute that he would only venture beyond the admission ward if driven to do so in order to protect his back, and in the expectation of finding some breach of regulations. These breaches were usually imaginary, but he was quite capable of haring off with all the zeal of a dedicated witch-hunter if he suspected he could create some ground for complaint. Once, for a full week, we were reduced to having only one full-time medical officer and an elderly half-timer to undertake night duties and on-call duties out of hours (the two consultants did not demean themselves with routine visits). In mid-week, George rang me up, peremptory and exasperated. It had come to his attention that a particular ward of elderly people had not seen a doctor on the previous day: perhaps I would arrange for someone to undertake daily visits of all wards. Since there were 15 wards in all, his request revealed such a grotesque failure to grasp the practical realities of the situation that there was really no room for irritation, and certainly not for rational discussion. I asked him who he could suggest to make up the shortfall of staff; he simply replaced his receiver.

His deputy was forward-looking, with liberal pretensions, a genial man who fraternised freely with all the staff. He saw the place as a community, and was inclined to indulge himself with slightly wild psychoanalytic ideas. He did have the faintly smug self-assurance of someone who is deeply confident of his own rectitude, and if one were tactless enough to imply any criticism at all of his judgements, he could respond with all the ruthless coldness of the analyst whose interpretation has been called in question. Brian, however, was serving his time until he took up a post in a prestigious institution in the south of England, and after a few weeks he left to occupy a position where he could spread his wings to better effect.

Ted, Brian's successor, was a man George had known a few years before, and no doubt George felt secure in having obtained the services of someone who could be relied upon not to rock the boat of biological orthodoxy.

For a little while, Ted, in his first consultancy, sat dutifully at the feet of his mentor, attentively soaking up George's grandiose plans for a well-run modern hospital. It was not very long, however, before Ted showed his true colours. He was at heart a swashbuckling buccaneer of a man who was perfectly capable of upsetting anybody's best-laid schemes. Ted, indeed, revelled in setting cats among pigeons, and did so consistently and unpredictably for the next 25 years.

His forte was a capacity for immediacy of action, which he combined with a certain inventiveness of technique and a general exuberant display of energy that was distinctly breathtaking. He combined this with a phenomenal flair for knowing the topic of the day in a specialty which was on the verge of expanding beyond recognition. Government reports were his bread and butter: Seebohm (social workers), Salmon (nursing structures), Trethowan (psychologists) and heaven knows what else, all became topics which he could bandy around committee tables with the greatest deftness and agility. I once saw him introduce a totally extraneous item into a completely unrelated agenda; he did so with such verve that everybody listened to him attentively and patiently while he bubbled away through a long and entirely irrelevant account of doings that were quite unconnected with our business.

He also had a knack of finding highly dramatic social problems; many years after the event, one of his nurses gave me a garbled account of an occasion when Ted precipitately admitted a couple who had apparently suffered a threefold disaster – let us say, an accidental death, substantial destruction of the matrimonial home by fire and the imminence of proceedings for divorce. The features are fictitious, but the scale of Ted's operations could well have been of this order. It we imagine that the wife was mute and prostrate, and the husband homicidally frustrated, the picture would be in keeping.

It was also in keeping that the couple were discharged after one weekend in care. Somehow, nursing staff and social workers rose to the occasion, and the two days' break proved to be enough.

As the years went by, Ted opened one fashionably specialised unit after another – for children, for alcoholics, for day-patients, out-patients, anything – always without forward planning, totally without regard for revenue consequences or staffing requirements, or for anything except some disregarded space which could be turned opportunistically to good use.

Staff and management alike rose magnificently to each new challenge. Nurses revelled, wallowed even, in their new-found opportunities. Ultimately, the children's unit found a young, balanced, visionary man who welded the entire set-up into a harmonious, smoothly running whole. In a single building set apart from the rest, disturbed youngsters, untrained nurses, psychologists, social workers, teachers, physiotherapists, occupational therapists and a devoted secretary established a working entity of such endurance that it outlived the abysmal mêlée which in the end swept away in months the whole physical embodiment of a century's good intentions.

The children's unit, Poplar Cottage, found a small discarded local hospital not too far away and happily continued to flourish.

The alcoholic unit came to draw heavily on experience of

peer-group management and the dedication of one charge nurse, and it too flourished within the limits of its resources until the end came.

Day patient care degenerated into farce as ambulances ferried seeming hordes of patients from 30 miles around to arrive in time for lunch at an effectively horrendous public expense, in order to depart again shortly afterwards.

Out-patient sessions developed their own horrifying tempo: Ted had devised a treatment of his own deriving from the discovery that some people (usually in the armed forces) could be significantly helped if they were enabled to recover the memories of some event which they had been unable to live with. Sometimes this could be achieved by using suitable doses of drugs which would relax the effort of suppressing the relevant memories. Ted therefore took to using a small dose of short-acting anaesthetic by injection: this had the effect of inducing a short period of unconsciousness and relaxation. It was quick, cheap and safe. Ted had the audacity to confer upon it the name 'catharsis', and every Monday morning, queues of people would assemble to await their few minutes of convenient unconscious bliss.

This was all very well. By the time the fashion caught on, the hospital had had to engage numbers of part-time medical staff, all of them mature, intelligent people (some of them wives of professional men, some of them general practitioners) and they too queued and jostled to find a spare cubicle or a screen where they could provide their quick fix. What made the proceedings disagreeable for some of the staff was that electrical treatment was also given at the same time and in the same place (until, at least, a special annexe was built which had the advantage of making everything much more aesthetic for the staff, in terms of plate glass, chromium plate, pot plants and space to move around in).

The electrical treatment (abhorred by many analysts but a genuine life-saver for selected patients) was marginally more risky than the simple 'cathartic' injection, but it had the snag that each individual treatment, while normally uneventful, did require to be very diligently monitored throughout. This disadvantage, minor in itself, became compounded when 20 or 30 patients were involved in each session: only two rows of six beds were available, so that one had to work down one row and back along the next, with a couple of breaks in the morning's work. Since recovery was much more prolonged after this modified ECT, the proceedings as a whole became thoroughly tiresome. They constituted in effect something known to psychologists as a 'vigilance task' – that is to say, a long period of alertness for a rare event – something known to be fraught and wearisome.

What was almost worse was that people were selected for ECT purely on the say-so of their consultant. The team of half a dozen nurses and doctors were consequently committed to a long, dull, repetitious mechanical task demanding a constant high degree of awareness for people whose probable benefit they could not even guess at.

Add to all this the high probability that every doorway in sight would be occupied by a harassed part-timer clutching a syringe, swabs, ampoule and a small dish.... The very first fruits of promotion were to fall with liberation from the bondage of those Monday mornings.

After Brian left, it could be said that the medical direction of patient care ceased to exist, or even worse, that it became a virtue to reduce resident numbers quite without regard for their subsequent provision. Central government fostered the process by declaring that after 15 years there would be no further requirement for any long-stay beds; this was done by enlisting the aid of a statistician who noted the actual decline over a five-year period and made the grotesque assumption that the same reduction in numbers would continue each year (rather than the same *proportionate* reduction in numbers). Subsequent independent publications of the correct calculation were ignored. The headlong commitment to an imaginary ideal of 'scientific' omnipotence was not to be halted.

A few lame footnotes may be in order, in the light of subsequent developments. First, the wave of 'therapeutic furor' which swept psychiatrists in general towards an exclusive concentration on out-patients and short-term admission did not at once mean that hundreds of remaining residents fell into neglect. On the contrary, moderation of excessive enthusiasm for the 'medical model' meant that the collective wisdom of the nursing staff was able to exert itself with generally beneficial effects. This remark in turn deserves a comment or two on historical context.

The psychiatry which Western, economically thriving countries have come to accept is attributed (by one Aubrey Lewis) to an epiphany around 1790, with Tuke, Chiarugi (from Florence) and Pinel, thanks to whom the insane could finally be treated ' on medical rather than moral lines ... psychiatry was thus born'.[9] Porter himself remarks that Lewis's judgement seems downright perverse, given that William Tuke was not a medical man, and stressed moral rather than medical means. In fact the term 'psychiatry' (as 'psychiaterie') is said to date from 1845, and its first used in English, according to the magisterial *Oxford English Dictionary*, from 1890. Professor Lewis in any case had something of a reputation as a therapeutic nihilist, and was surely wrong to ignore the first and probably the finest example of 'community care' at Gheel in Belgium, which dates from medieval times. Henderson and Gillespie mention Gheel,[10] but it is ignored by nearly all writers in English.

Then again, Pinel, while an undoubted polymath, was not in good standing with the French medical establishment; his approach involved psychological techniques in place of accepted physical methods, and he did not himself do most of the work with patients: he preferred to remain apart while his lay superintendent, Pussin, dealt with the patients.[11] And medicine in general only intruded on the scene with the establishment of large asylums in the nineteenth century. The advent of pharmaceutical manufacturing on a large scale bids fair to undermine whatever contribution medicine ever made towards the existence of psychiatry.

The decay of what had once been a medical influence in psychiatry was modified at Brightways by one fortunate circumstance. This was the resonance, almost a distant drum-roll, of a psychoanalytic influence. By chance, a psychiatric social worker and a couple of mature, intelligent, sensitive married women who were part-time doctors had all sat at the feet of an analyst at the nearest medical school 60 miles away, and they were able to introduce a form of group therapy into the admission ward and the out-patient department, housed in its splendid new purpose-built annexe. 'Group discussions' might have been a more accurate description, but at all events the influence of peer groups proved inestimably beneficial. Even George, no longer so heavily burdened by his title of Superintendent, and feeling vastly less threatened by divergent opinions among his colleagues, succumbed to the benevolent ebb and flow of ideas which the groups introduced. His last years were free of the asperity, suspicion and persecution which had tormented him and his hospital at the outset.

Other factors too had begun to broaden the therapeutic base of the institution. Psychologists were appointed, and additional social workers. The nursing staff on the long-stay wards used their new initiative to organise a variety of outdoor activities by way of clearing undergrowth from local estates, reducing the dead wood to eminently saleable firewood, as well as by organising holiday periods to seaside resorts. Bearing in mind the dread image of the administrative staff, it has to be said that these large-scale activities, involving matters of staff allowances and overtime, as well as costs and benefits, did incur a deal of accurate and co-operative thinking on the part of grey-suited individuals normally thought of as confining their activities to the issue of stern and often obstructive memoranda.

Finally, Brightways did have one quality which I never observed anywhere else: I had been told that in any hospital (or any psychiatric hospital) there was an undying hostility between nursing staff and artisans – that is, the small army of engineers, painters, electricians, joiners and many others without whom the hospital could not exist. In part, this must have dated from the days when most large asylums were run by the local authority, and the artisan staff had an unwritten tradition of helping themselves discreetly to material benefits at public expense, before reasonable wages were paid after the introduction of the National Health Service. I never grasped anything like the full extent or the nature of this animosity, but its absence at Brightways was notable.

Many of the staff of this rural hospital were related either by blood or by marriage, often through two or three generations, and the resulting bonhomie must have done much to lend the place a feeling of solidarity almost to the end. This was illustrated by an incident which also illuminated the profound (and understandable) bitterness that existed between the hospital secretary and the clinical staff.

The secretary, one Morphy, was an incomer. He kept himself to himself and enjoyed the use of the most spacious office in the building. Entry was rarely permitted and truth to tell was always a pleasure. He was a first-rate administrator who had the highly unenviable task of mediating between a management committee which seemed invariably to be both wantonly authoritarian and thoroughly wayward on the one hand, and medical and nursing staff on the other who were unaccountable to anyone, and not just capricious but consistently and infuriatingly arrogant to boot.

It is not surprising then that on the rare occasions when he found the chance, he leapt at any opportunity of besting the clinical staff with all the vigour at his command, and without the least shred of compunction.

For instance, in some remote corner of the kingdom there had been allegations of neglect by nursing staff which had attracted national publicity. Fred Morphy then set himself with superlative craftsmanship to put together a document for strictly limited circulation among the clerical and artisan staffs. This document contrived to forge, in straight, simple English, an invitation to the 'lay' staff of the hospital to report to him any abuse of residents (patients) which they might see, but its artistry lay in the way this was put together in such a manner that it gave no opportunity at all for offence if by any mischance it should fall into wrong hands.

It happened that one of the nursing staff managed to 'borrow' a copy of this seditious document and produce a small number of copies, which were quietly circulated among his chosen cronies. I was on good terms with the crafty, villainous Bill, who let me have a copy of my own, which I nursed carefully in a secret drawer.

Needless to say, Fred's exercise was quite pointless, but it did throw into relief the solidarity among all the staff which still existed at the time. For all I know, Bill's exercise may have been quite unnecessary, but it transpired that a particularly thoughtful and responsible nurse was making his way one day down a deserted corridor when he heard from above him the call of a cheerful and amiable voice: 'Watch it, Rick, we've got our eye on you!' It was a painter, far above among the timbers of the roof.

In such an atmosphere, there could be no great cause for concern.

Unavoidably, among two or three hundred people in such a close community, there were currents and counter-currents, but they were mostly among people of the same grade, and mostly too they were part and parcel of common gossip.

If, as it seemed to me, the medical direction of the hospital was at best vacuous and at worst perverse, the extensive sense of kinship which pervaded the place as a whole must have done a great deal to hold it together and keep it functioning until the higher levels of political administration finally made it unworkable.

Before the advent of tranquillising drugs, a report of the World Health Organisation appeared, bearing on the subject of mental hospitals in general. Its authors declared in a passing expression of sagacity that the quality of an institution could be gauged in passing from the front gates towards the main door. On this criterion, Brightways would have passed muster. The main driveway was short, straight, and led through a large open forecourt directly to the modest reception area. On the way one passed a small, expensive and incongruously unobtrusive piece of modern sculpture which had been commissioned to commemorate the centenary of the establishment. Within the small reception area, one wall sported an unpretentious bronze plaque, also commemorating the centenary. This plaque was normally illuminated by an appropriately small overhead light; each night when the receptionist went home, her last ritual duty was to switch off this light and to draw a pair of tiny curtains in order to conceal the (frankly rather splendid) bit of bronze: all this strictly ordained by the magnificently punctilious secretary, whose consistent obsessionality was put to vastly more creative purposes than that of the fussy and ineffectual George.

In fact, the approach and surroundings of the hospital were so agreeable as to go a long way towards compensating for the horrors of working there. At any rate, the judgement of the World Health Organisation's report may have been more far-sighted than mine. One last memory may serve to suggest that it was; after long years, the ultimate promotion came my way, and with it a thoroughly healthy measure of independence, not to mention the services of a personal typist and the use of a cosy little office handily placed close to the main entrance. Now and again I left my little office to go home a little later than usual, when the hospital was quiet, the residents fed, the day shift preparing to go off duty, and just a couple of cleaners pottering about near the small entrance hall. They were a cheerful couple, and we usually exchanged a few friendly words before I walked out past the reception desk.

The receptionists too were all models of their kind. Unassuming, well-informed and helpful (as they should be!), they too were always good for a brief exchange of news at the end of the day. If there had to be a last view of Brightways, this easy, relaxed atmosphere, embracing all grades and functions regardless of rank or seniority, could have been symbolic of a kind of unity I had not seen elsewhere. If the place seemed to lack any overall purpose other than its own destruction, and even if bitterness, malice and frank ill will found small sectarian pockets in which to flourish, there was to the very end an underlying current of familiarity which a larger, better, bigger institution would have lacked. Of the years I spent there, many were frustrating and many unrewarding; it was still among the very few bodies whose reunions I was glad to attend after its final decline and fall.

7

Patients

When the charitable ideals of Victorian England proved to have ground to a halt, and before any kind of scientific approach had begun to pay dividends, there was on the whole little for the more thoughtful English psychiatrist to do but to speculate on the psychological theories originating in Vienna: for about 30 years, these seemed to be ideally suited to the economic and intellectual climate of the times. Popular accounts of psychoanalysis appeared to offer a systematic approach to the understanding and relief of the lesser degrees of disturbed behaviour and personal suffering. But the endless duplicities of language have seen to it not only that schisms appeared almost from the first in the 'scientific' aspirations of psychoanalysis, but also that the 'happy sphere of one-to-one familiar address', the 'springs of authentic human understanding'[12], slip away inescapably through the words (between the lines as it were) of theoretical formulations. So it is that the nature of the therapeutic encounter between two people not only escapes logical formulation, but has also spread unavoidably into spheres of activity which could never have been envisaged among the fringes of neurological practice, steeped in the growing positivism of early scientific hopes in Middle Europe.

So, too, the jargon of psychoanalysis has gained footholds far and wide among Western thought, often sadly with the dreadful results which follow when a new algorithm (a new 'decision procedure') appears to present itself; that is to say, that ill-defined and insufficiently explored realities are made to fit some rigid, narrow form of words which crowds out the spontaneous, the novel and the creative.

For my part, I had entered psychiatry with the advantage of having stood in need of help myself, and of having had the benefit of some experience on the couch, which bolstered my thirst for sound theorising with enough practical experience to be useful.

Nothing can quite evoke the experience of personal analysis, and while the techniques of therapy on this basis may all exist within a common framework, any technique is always put to use by some particular unique individual: 'technique' of its own can produce only an empty brilliance. Behind technique there has to be room for countless infinities of discovery; for discovery and for surprise. So an enterprise based on an analytic approach has to be one of endless patience and of great vigilance. One distinguished analyst declared roundly that 'the analyst who is not surprised by his patient's productions or by his own reactions is not doing his job properly'. (All discussions on technique in therapy always seem to involve quirky personal observations in the nature of *obiter dicta* – sayings by the wayside – and I think that this is as true of surgery, say, or of painting, composing or building, as it is of the apparently formal encounter in a psychological setting.)

In any case, the demands of a public service in provincial practice do place stringent limits on what can and what has to be done: what passes for 'therapy' under these conditions can only amount to a small portion of one's time. Even remembering that the term 'therapeutic institution' was invented in 1943, and gained widespread currency in the English-speaking world, it was perhaps more honoured by lip-service than in concrete terms – yet the idea was there as an ideal to aim for, and in the hands of men like Ian Pearson it did, for a while, embody some heady aspirations in a number of enlightened institutions.

But my own interests lay in the exploration of the person-to-person encounter, and if my formal skills were limited, now and again they proved to be well adapted to circumstance.

What delighted me most was to find now and then that someone, some 'patient', some 'client', could reach a point at which they would say, 'Well, that's it then; I've had enough – it's been nice to know you, but I'll manage on my own from now on.'

I found this uniquely gratifying. Whether or not it meant that my opposite number – my patient, my client, that person – had finally come to feel that I had no more to offer, or whether indeed they had gained enough to become truly independent, I do not know. Possibly the two points of view amount in the end to the same thing – that one has fulfilled the role of a 'good enough' parent figure.

An end result like this could come about in different ways. Sometimes there was no ending, just a gradually increasing familiarity with a situation, a problem, an individual, until the frequency of visits decreased, or the force of events brought about a rupture for external reasons.

On one splendid occasion, a dignified professional gentleman came to see me with a specific difficulty; he was a well-educated man, thoroughly amiable, and we got on together splendidily. I decided (rightly, I am sure) that a head-on onslaught would prove to be quite unprofitable, and week after week we spent the time discussing various apparently peripheral difficulties in his life (as well as some delights), always in the most agreeable and cultivated way. After a year or so, I felt it was time that we returned to our muttons, and I put the matter to him point-blank.

'By the way,' I said, 'what about the old problem?'

He laughed. 'Oh, that!' he said. 'That cleared up months ago!'

I have forgotten what arrangements we came to thereafter, or rather I do remember that he had achieved promotion, which meant a welcome move (for him) to the other end of the country. Conceivably it was that prospect which helped him to overcome the trouble he had presented me with. One really never knows.

Very occasionally, it was possible to find dramatic results with minimum effort. One such result came about with a young woman who presented with sudden onset of what sounded like a form of agoraphobia. She was a bright, beautifully turned-out woman, and a thoroughly personable individual. She had recently married a man of Czech origins, and since Slavonic family names normally vary with gender, I thought to trip her up by asking why she used the male form of her husband's name. The answer was very simple: she was English, and she followed the English fashion of using her husband's name.

This slightly puerile exchange laid the basis for a good working relationship, and we set to work to establish the facts of the case, which were purely and simply that since her marriage she had developed a crippling dread of driving her car. This was odd, she said, because previously she had enjoyed using the full potential of a particularly agile little sports car.

At this, the coincidence of her marriage with the onset of her inhibition struck me with special force, and I made a thoroughly ill-judged comment to the effect that she had previously been a fast young woman and was now respectably married. It was a perfect example of a sound interpretation with exquisitely bad timing, and it left her completely nonplussed, as it deserved to. (This was not, I must say, a mistake that I made a habit of.)

As before, it was very clear that a head-on onslaught was pointless, and we spent some time discussing the circumstances of her work, her employer, and other matters of general interest.

Before long, she turned up for her appointment with the news that on the previous Saturday night she had run out of cigarettes, and she had felt obliged to take her car (by this time a modest family saloon) for half a mile down the road to the nearest off-licence, travelling all the way in bottom gear, very slowly, and keeping close to the kerb all the way.

From then on she made steady progress, step by step, entirely under her own initiative, for all the world as though some invisible psychologist had taken her through a graded exercise of increasing difficulty. The following week she reported with glee that she had repeated her journey and had found it necessary on the way to overtake a pedal-cyclist. Her ability to do this came as a genuine surprise. A week later, she had been able to travel in second gear, and for a slightly longer journey. And so it went on, until within a few weeks she was completely recovered. I had never seen anything like this: phobias were generally quite intractable to treat, though it is true that they usually take a much more chronic form, and only turn up in the consulting-room after many years of incapacity. Perhaps at least I had made available for Peggy some little measure of space, time and security, with enough sympathetic yet disinterested attention (always prime ingredients) to enable her to come to terms with part of her real self.

Two men who showed quite a different resolution to their problems were among a select handful for whom I set aside one evening a week. This provided longer sessions than were possible in the ordinary crowded clinics in the local general hospitals.

One of these was an intelligent man with a middling job in the Civil Service, where failure to seek promotion was considered to be a significant short-coming. Tom's particular position was one grade below a level which was known to have broken three men in the immediate district, and he knew quite realistically that his memory was not up to coping with the vast amounts of highly detailed regulations which promotion would involve.

He ascribed his inadequate memory to experiences in childhood which he remembered quite clearly: his mother (of whom he had no distinct recollection as an individual) had disappeared under circumstances which were as distressing to his father as her unforeseen absence was to him. His father therefore had constantly drummed into him that 'the past is a closed book – forget it'.

This instruction, handed down from on high, had come to haunt him, and when he saw a particularly vivid demonstration of hypnotic regression on one of the ever-intrusive television slots, he conceived of an immediate answer to his situation – recourse to a quite unusually deep level of hypnosis.

We must have discussed this for a while, and eventually I spent half an hour with him, trying to get him to relax and to induce a light hypnoidal trance. He went through the motions reasonably enough, and when he opened his eyes again, I suggested that he might profitably practise relaxation in his own home.

At this he grunted, and moped a little. 'Aargh,' he said, 'you mean I have to inflict this on myself on top of everything else?'

Well, no, but come and see me again and we'll see what we can do.

So he did come, quite regularly for months on end, and we explored his many woes and his few pleasures at some length. As usual, his immediate preoccupations were quite other than the one which had prompted his referral. We chatted away quite happily for session after session, with some breaks for dramatic changes in his lifestyle (as when he decided to leave his family and take bachelor quarters for a while) until one dark evening he arrived and slumped in the one available armchair, a picture of abject misery. I was frankly alarmed, and penned a hasty letter for his own doctor, recommending a potent antidepressant preparation. He came again the following week, and for half an hour he poured out a morose catalogue of his current tribulations. When he finished, I was keen to find out if he had been taking the medicine, and asked him directly.

'Ah, no,' he replied, and without the least change in his demeanour he added blandly that he had decided that from thenceforth he would look after his own problems. There was no rancour and no sense of disillusion behind his decision; just a bald statement of fact.

This was not quite the reasoned and well-considered announcement which (on the occasions that it happened) I found so uniquely gratifying. Nor by any means had he been transformed into a ball of fire. We did in fact meet again, more than five years later, and then only for him to confirm a decision he had made in respect of another member of his family who was then consulting me. He was still the same plain-spoken undistinguished man he had always been, except that now his decisions were decisions, and his tolerance for a life of quiet desperation considerably increased.

For years after he stopped his regular visits I wondered if my alarm at his state of depression had convinced him that I acted in good faith, and had been enough to persuade him that he could go it alone. Now I am not so sure, and I would have to rephrase my thoughts in much more arcane terms, which would make for a different kind of work.

The other chap who belonged among my 'Tuesday specials' was, superficially at least, quite a different character. He had a uniformly lugubrious appearance, and had acquired the habit of finding the company of women who were socially speaking available, but so intimidating to him that he lived in a perpetual muck sweat of indecision with each new potential companion.

It is true that in the long run he did find a patient, faithful young widow who would gladly have taken him into her home. The snag in her case was that she had a couple of young children, who provided the perfect excuse for his prevarication. Their association was nevertheless constant and enduring enough to present a considerable improvement on his previous dithering, and to this extent the outcome should have been gratifying. It is true too that in the end he also made the decision to go his own way. It was almost as though, in the jargon, he had managed to internalise a good enough object to enable him to stand on his own feet. He expressed this in a slightly peculiar way by saying that as long as he knew that I would be available on the end of a telephone, he would be content. There was something slightly creepy and unwholesome about him, or about our relationship, and truth to tell I remember him best perhaps for something trivial in itself, yet which might have represented a critical moment on his path.

It happened that before he settled down with his faithful Mary, he had developed a passion (one among many other bizarre and deeply ambivalent fancies) for a woman who worked at the counter of a local multiple store which was within easy walking distance of the office where he worked. He therefore had the option of going along during his lunch-hour on the chance that he would be able to talk to his latest lady-love, but he knew that he also stood the risk of being given, in plain English, a pretty brisk brush-off. During one of his sessions, he agonised about this situation at some length, and finally turned his despairing eyes in my direction to plead for a decision. Should he or shouldn't he (and he enlarged yet again on the oh so finely balanced possibilities of exquisite delight and intolerable rebuff)? Should he? Or should he not? His baleful glare swivelled again in my direction. This was, of course, strictly against the rules. His decisions were to be his own decisions: my part was to 'keep the heid' and calmly present him with a suitably digestible version of his position. Conceivably that is what I did, though that is not what it felt like at the time. I felt instead both angry and irritated, and I turned upon him with some deliberation.

Of what use, I asked him, would any decision of mine be to him? In either case he would remain wretched and dissatisfied (and it was now my turn to enlarge upon his own exposition of his dilemma, which I did at some length). The longer I spoke, the more he paid attention, until finally we had both had enough, and the time came for his visit to draw to an end.

His eyes shining, I escorted him the few paces down the corridor to the front door of the building. As we approached the reception area he turned to face me, his face alight, and he embarked upon a profuse expression of thanks. I had not spared him, he said; I had given him the plain unvarnished truth, and he appreciated it – and some more of the like.

To this day I cannot altogether account for his reaction. I saw it once, much later, under quite different circumstances, and found it equally astonishing. Possibly he too, like his forgetful predecessor, had detected something more than a mere couch-side manner, which had given him a degree of confidence that he could make his own.

Perhaps one needs to have not only some capacity to provide a measure of space, time and security, but also some capacity too for the incalculable, the ineffable ability now and again to be able to find a deeply felt human response which will be appropriate to the occasion.

* * *

One woman, more than anybody else, seemed to respond ideally to my own personal mix of abilities.

She was a modest, quietly spoken woman in early middle life; her speech was always restrained but clear, and her invariable candour made my part of our work so much the easier.

Her symptoms, too, were rather vague: she felt herself to be severely incapacitated, but without any of the regular, dramatic textbook signs of inexplicable weeping, loss of appetite, inability to sleep, bouts of panic and so forth. Nevertheless, in her own quiet and firmly stated (even understated) way, she had become completely unable to conduct her normal life to her own satisfaction. Her husband, it is true, had been made redundant, and she herself was unable to follow her own modest job as a cleaner, but her husband was able to do enough part-time work as a jobbing gardener to meet their needs. They were able to keep their elderly motor car on the road, though she herself was no longer able to drive it about. Her one son maintained his own family without impinging unduly on her own, and while her husband's shortage of work was a worry, her anxieties on that score seemed to be well within the limits of what would be normal.

We spent some months gently exploring her family background and the development of her disability; in fact, it was quite a long time before I felt able to probe at all in that area, or she, for her part, able to tell me about it. It transpired that her incapacity had been precipitated by a ludicrously trivial accident on a quiet country road when a careless bicyclist had driven into her car, without any serious damage to either of the vehicles or of their owners.

She was quite clear about this incident and its importance in reducing her to a nervous wreck, but for weeks before this emerged in the course of our conversations, she had been preoccupied by the circumstances of her upbringing.

She had been brought up by rather elderly grandparents in a particularly remote country cottage. It took her some time to explain that her grandparents had not been in any way cruel or unkind, at least in any conventional sense, but it was clear that by reason of their age, their social isolation and their adherence to a rigidly puritanical lifestyle, they had been quite unable to provide the warmth and liveliness which a young girl could reasonably expect.

How this came about was never made clear in precise terms; possibly the harsh realities of life had forced the situation upon them, since she came to know her natural mother perfectly well long before her school-days were over, and accepted her precisely as she accepted any other of the familiar figures in the local township, and with no more feeling either of warmth or of distance than she felt for any other of the townsfolk – of whom, of course, she saw very little in any case.

By the time all this had been made clear, I felt able to ask about her contacts with friends at school. There was no problem. She had plenty of friends at the school. Boyfriends? By now she was able to giggle a little in her own reserved fashion. Yes, yes, plenty of boyfriends.

Yet this little giggle foreshadowed more than I could have guessed at. A week or two later, with no preamble at all, she declared in her own quiet forthright way that for two full years before she saw me, she had lived in a nightmarish state which she could not convey in words.

I turned back through her notes to verify the date when I had first seen her, and my impression of her at that time: while I was doing this, she added that her distress had been so great as to make her contemplate suicide.

At this I was distinctly startled, and remarked that she had not said so at the time. She agreed, and added that she had not told her family doctor either. Then she chuckled again at the memory, and added, 'I took very good care not to!'

From this point onwards, everything was plain sailing. Her conversation turned much more towards current preoccupations and future prospects, though we were not yet quite out of the woods. Shortly afterwards, her husband found a regular job with prospects of a permanent appointment, and an occupational pension at the end of it. This involved moving house a distance of ten miles or so across country, but she continued to make the more difficult journey by bus to see me regularly.

Then her son was made redundant, and moved into his mother's home until he was able to stand on his own feet again. Cynthia now became somewhat irritable, even petulant. After a few weeks it was clear that in fact her son as well as his wife with two young children and most of his furniture were all sharing her small three-bedroomed house. Her worries now were much more transparent and appropriate to the realities of the situation.

Fortunately, this extremely wearing burden did resolve itself, and our appointments gradually became less frequent, until one month, with Christmas approaching, it seemed reasonable to allow a longer gap than usual, and I blandly asked her if another session three months away would be agreeable.

She was distinctly put out at this idea. 'Do I really have to come again? The bus services are really very awkward.'

Of course she was right. Her husband's move had meant that she had to take an infrequent country service for five miles in the opposite direction in order to catch a bus to bring her ten miles back again to the clinic. It seemed clear that I had served my purpose. She was not bored, her visits had not been pointless, but our joint efforts had been successful, and it was quite unrealistic to make the long cold journey for the sake of a now merely conversational break in her normal daily routine.

I could not have wished a more businesslike conclusion to our efforts.

* * *

No one should imagine that psychiatry was ever all about listening, patience and understanding. Indeed, if there were ever some systematic exposition of what it was all about, it would, I am sure, be bound to miss some point at some stage, if only because it is in the nature of living things to have indeterminacy built in. It would be agreeable to explore this quasi-mystical, unforeseeable background at much greater length, but the cost is too high and the prospects too few to make it rewarding.

Just the same, it seems worthwhile to include a history to illustrate both sides of the coin – the personal and the systematic – if only because in the end the business of living is not so much about 'either/or' as about 'both/and'.

One man more than any other fills the bill. He came to see me at about the age of sixty, after a few years of retirement from a professional position in the armed forces.

He had been, let us say, an expert in signalling and electronics, and he had gained a respectable rank as well as being very actively involved with the day-to-day business of armed combat. He had the advantage, then, of a stable and cultivated background, which made both his acquaintance and the management of his problems so much the more tractable.

His story, on the face of it, was quite straightforward. From the age of forty he had begun to suffer from episodes of depression which little by little had become increasingly severe and increasingly frequent. At first they had no doubt responded to such measures as medicine could offer, or they had perhaps been subject to 'spontaneous remission'. He came to see me during one of these periods of remission, which certainly made for a good start in terms of history-taking and general appraisal of the situation. We began with a routine approach of gentle exploration of problems, origins and general background. For some time all went well, until one day he turned up looking quite unable to cope, harassed and demoralised, and deserving, I felt, a trial with a first-line preparation of an antidepressant.

We got the dose right first time, and when he showed signs of a good recovery after a few weeks, we were able to taper off his dosage bit by bit without any immediate recurrence of his disturbance.

For a good few months, all remained well, until one fine day he arrived looking sufficiently agitated and dejected as to deserve something rather more potent than he had had before. Accordingly, he agreed to take a preparation which, while usually more effective, was also customarily used with more circumspection than the ordinary run-of-the-mill product which he had had the first time.

Once again, we hit on the right dosage; in a few weeks he made a good recovery yet again, and a gradual reduction of his dose produced not the least sign of any untoward reaction.

This time he remained well for nearly a full year, but his next relapse struck just as suddenly as the others, and with even greater force. This time his condition of abject incoherence called, I felt, for nothing less than full-blown electrical treatment. Jack retained enough independence of mind to refuse admission to hospital, and one of his family agreed to run him back and forth on alternate weekdays in order to let him have the treatment as an out-patient. A conventional course lasts for a fortnight, or six doses; after three applications, Jack was considerably improved, and agreed with some reluctance to one further visit to the main hospital. This fourth visit proved quite sufficient, and he had no further problems from that time onwards.

This pattern of depression, with late onset and gradually increasing severity of attacks, is quite an unusual one. At first, I was inclined to remember Jack as a man who illustrated the virtues of both the 'medical model' of psychiatry, (a.k.a. the 'pills-and-potions' approach) and of such skill in the ineffable art of 'dynamic psychology' (a.k.a. 'depth psychology' or even 'couch-side manner') as I could muster. Looking back, I am inclined to wonder whether the essentially permissive approach which I adopted had not allowed him for the first time to reveal more and more about a problem which was more deeply rooted than he had let himself (or anyone else) be aware of previously. To this extent, he could have belonged with my two 'Tuesdays specials', who, I guessed, required a genuine, spontaneous display of interest before they felt secure enough to face the world on their own.

In Jack's case, I was lucky to have the resources of contemporary pharmacy available (as well as ECT), since, if my guess is right, the revelation of a full-blown depression would have required months or even years of extremely patient nursing care. On the other hand, Jack's position may have been rather different. Our conversations nearly always turned on his current working life. He had a profitable hobby which gave him plenty to talk about, as well as for me to listen to (he was neither a bore nor a fanatic). His martial reminiscences were also freely available on request, but any enquiry about his family life was inclined to get short shrift. I wonder now whether his capacity for moving successfully in professional spheres in male company may not have required more of his attention than was entirely healthy. He was not of an age when he would have much opportunity for any radical change in his personal approach to life, but then he never showed any sign of the kind of personal problems in relation to other people which are evident in patients with whom I could successfully adopt a psychological approach along mainly permissive and generally non-interventionist lines. Jack's treatment turned out on the face of it to have been palliative – but then, palliation of one distress does sometimes allow another more creative capacity to flourish.

Which thought makes for not only a mulberry bush of intractable size, but perhaps also for a burning bush of impenetrable illumination. At least, the extraordinary interplay of personal, social, technical, economic and even of random influences which are all visible to the informed observer of the scene may go some way to illustrating my own admittedly rather dismissive remark to Professor David's wife – yes, psychiatry does have its excitements, but yes, indeed it can be a very bizarre kind of discipline.

The fashions of today require neat, theoretical explanations to lend credibility to our actions: to explode this idea would take a learned tome – a whole series of learned tomes – and it would still involve a mass of anecdotal evidence. Yet what else do we live by? In my closing chapters, I shall have to resort, *faute de mieux*, to such anecdotes as I can muster in order to paint a thin wash of background for the picture which lies in the foreground of memory. Scholarly hands are at work these days constructing histories of psychiatry which are mostly more notable for their academic credentials than for any great conviction in terms of everyday life.

At some point, Freud saw fit to quote Goethe: '*Grau ist alle*

Theorie, mein Freund; grün das Lebens ewige Baum' (All theory is grey, my friend; green the ever-living tree of Life). So a few stray leaves from the dark forest of life will have to serve, like Andrew Collins's aspidistra, to enliven the passing scene.

8

Nurses

The first hospital in England to be founded specifically for the care of the disturbed was built in 1713 as a private house and bequeathed in 1724 'for the reception and habitation of poor lunatics...'[13] Patricia Allderidge adds that the hospital, though apparently acceptable to God, to Whom it was dedicated, did not meet the more stringent requirements of the Department of Health, and by 1978 was already unlikely to survive in a recognisable form.

In 1728, Guy's Hospital in London was founded for incurables, with specific provision in the will of its founder for incurable lunatics, and a separate 'lunatic house' was duly built. (Bethlem, very much older, was not founded originally to house lunatics specifically, and while it must have been the first public hospital for the insane poor in England, a condition of entry was the supposition of cure within 12 months, when patients were discharged if they were not indeed cured.) In 1733, Bethlem in fact added accommodation for 100 incurables, and in 1751 a second specialised public hospital for the insane was founded in London by public subscription, and a lunatic hospital in Manchester opened in 1766. About the same time, a 'Hospital for Lunaticks' opened in Newcastle, and Hereford also acquired a public asylum. York opened an asylum in 1777, and Leicester added an asylum to its County Infirmary in 1794.

Finally, in 1807, a Parliamentary Select Committee sat to enquire into the state of pauper lunatics in England and

Wales, and the following year an Act was passed empowering the counties of England and Wales to establish public asylums; in 1845 these establishments were made mandatory.

The Select Committee of 1807 found that pauper lunatics who were detained under existing legislation were mostly in 'houses of correction', or in poorhouses or workhouses, or boarded out in private madhouses.

The Acts of 1808 and 1845, which first empowered and then required the construction of county asylums in England and Wales, were framed in optimistic terms. One has to wonder why, unless it were the case that private madhouses had shown themselves capable of managing small numbers of selected patients on the basis of private fees.

Parliament could not have foreseen the size of the demand for public asylums, nor the problems of running them at public expense. Yet the insufficiency of the number of keepers was recognised by the Parliamentary Committee of 1815 as one of the major deficiencies which afflicted existing madhouses.

The county asylums of England and Wales seem to have been doomed from the start. Their construction appears to have been intended to provide a material basis, in architectural terms, for management which had no systematic body of practice to draw on. Consequently the managers, at first, seem to have been a motley crew of civic worthies, and the actual keepers to have been drawn from the lower ranks of domestic servants, labourers and poor craftsmen. The turnover of staff was sometimes very high, most male attendants remaining for a matter of months only, and females perhaps a year or two.

Their duties were mainly domestic and menial, the hours long, and discipline very rigorous. The ratio of staff to inmates was very low (about 1 in 14), and training non-existent until 1890.[14,15]

Under such circumstances it is miraculous that a corps of experienced people should have emerged to staff the psychiatric hospitals through the twentieth century within traditions which often ran through three generations of a family, and embraced an unwritten expertise in the ways of disturbed individuals which could surpass the ability of most medical men and sometimes match that of the best of them.

The transition from 'keeper' to 'attendant' (asylum attendant, or attendant upon the insane) through to 'psychiatric nurse' is not an easy one for the outsider to trace. Formally, the term 'attendant' was in use in 1884, and the term 'mental nurse' officially used from 1919, but there were subtle, liberalising changes taking place which helped to transform the 'keepers' of the early nineteenth century into the loyal and dedicated body of people who became the psychiatric nurses of the twentieth. Night nurses were introduced, some leisure facilities provided for, and communal activities inaugurated which helped to foster some *esprit de corps* among the staff. Hospital bands and sports teams were already common by the end of the century, and gave rise to regular fixtures with other institutions (sometimes, as we have seen, involving needle matches with neighbouring establishments).

Initially, relations between the sexes on the staff had been proscribed under pain of dismissal, but it has to be borne in mind that the keepers of the early 1800s were almost as much confined to the premises as the inmates were. Inevitably, there came a time when marriages took place and, particularly in the smaller and more rural establishments, family traditions were established which proved to be widespread and durable.

By 1911, proposals had been made for asylum attendants to be pensionable, and it became possible (admittedly with some difficulty) to conceive of the asylum attendant as having, potentially at least, a lifelong career. In 1919 a special register for qualified attendants was established, when the term 'mental nurse' was also officially introduced.

The way forward, in terms of promotion, must have been difficult and uncertain. A charge nurse had an almost absolute sway over his ward. The routine of the day was spelt out hour by hour: even the physical disposition of the staff depended upon questions of seniority, and the work must often have been both frustrating and demanding. And it could be dangerous.

On the very night before I joined the staff of the Observation Unit, a young student nurse had been attacked by a patient because of a trivial misunderstanding in the darkness of the ward. The girl was not seriously hurt, but she was shaken enough to call for a sober, reflective comment from some of the more experienced staff.

'Well then, but everyone gets attacked – *once*.'

A little later, in the same hospital, a more experienced nurse was also attacked by mistake under similar circumstances, when a Polish patient, known to side with the staff, came to the rescue of the threatened man and misidentified his quarry. The nurse, a qualified and well-regarded individual, lost part of his ear as the result of a vigorous bite. The missing portion of the ear lobe was never found, despite a most diligent search. But the next morning, that nurse was despatched for immediate attention by the most noted cosmetic surgeon of the city, with firm recommendations as to the quality of care required.

Fatalities too were reported, but they were rare, and they always seemed to happen in benighted, previously unheard of parts of the country, a great distance away.

Yet in spite of everything, psychiatric nursing became a calling which could involve two or three generations of the same family. More than this, there were men who came to the job in the years of the depression simply to have a job, and who made a positive decision that once being in, they would make that their life's work. One of the Jims at Ramscar told me as much one afternoon with a quiet emphasis which was enormously impressive. He ran a ward almost single-handed, and his qualities were characteristic of the best of the male nurses. (The women's qualities seemed to sit more naturally with their gender: like the men, their abilities varied quite widely – the one thing that marked them out was a notable capacity for making a ward much more decorative and homely.)

Charge nurses in particular seemed to develop into the figure of the gentle giant. They were large men because from time to time an element of physical strength could be necessary, yet nearly all displayed a quality of reserve, a quietness of speech and a frugal use of words which could be most agreeable to work with. The more conservative could exert a deadening effect on the small changes of routine which might have transformed the frankly dreary lives of their charges; the Jim of whom I speak now was not such a man.

His ward was adjacent to what I suppose could have been called a 'refractory ward', let us say one of the more disturbed wards, where a degree of noisy and unpredictable behaviour could be expected more or less constantly. Jim's ward was never noisy, yet nor was it by any means a haven of rest. Indeed, part of it was a verandah, formerly used for tuberculous patients, which was currently supposed to represent the ultimate sanction that Ramscar could offer, in that men who supposedly could not be housed elsewhere were kept in bed on this verandah until they were deemed to have recovered enough equanimity to be up and about.

A parenthesis has to intrude at this point, since Ramscar, at any rate during my time, had no padded rooms whatever, and the only drugs then available as a drastic last resource would have been dangerous if used for more than short periods at a time. (In fact, it was on Jim's ward that I learned the value of using, on occasion, the very combination of morphia and hyoscine which the nursing staff at Hillside were to baulk at.) The point is that the padded room, when it comes to practicalities, was a comfortable, hygienic, almost cosy provision. One might say without being altogether too fanciful that it had some womblike properties, and it has been claimed that the majority of patients who used one did so at their own request. (This has the ring of truth about it: people do value their security, even when it implies drastic curtailment of their liberties.)

Jim's verandah, then, contained a dozen or so patients, all in bed, most of them for short periods of time until some acute period of disturbance had safely passed.

One of these men deserves a small deviation of the narrative to himself. This man was nursed entirely naked. Received wisdom had it that he would not tolerate clothing of any kind. Certainly when I first met him he had been nursed in this way for many months, and possibly for a year or more. I am sure that this account of him was accurate at the time: it was certainly consistent with his general demeanour. He was undoubtedly schizophrenic, but a vocal and relatively coherent schizophrenic. Quite soon after I met him he called out that he wanted to go home. Of course he did. But when he declared that he wanted his father and his mother, I felt that he had gone too far, and in an effort to reconcile him to his current situation, I made the rejoinder that for the time being, Dr Mack was his father and his mother. This struck home; for weeks thereafter, I had only to pass the foot of his bed for him to grumble away *sotto voce* in a disgusted kind of way, 'Dr Mack, father and mother, *hah.*' What became of him subsequently will soon appear.

The quality of Jim's personal commitment to his service became clear when he pointed out to me one day, quietly and with complete discretion, a man who had been held to be unmanageable outside the 'refractory' ward. This man had been moved back again to Jim's care because, as Jim said, 'he knows that I shall keep an eye on him.'

The fact of the matter was that the patient knew that he could not control his own impulses towards violence, and that, for that matter, neither would the regime in the disturbed ward be sufficient to do so. But he did know that Jim would give him enough personal attention to make sure that he behaved himself. He valued Jim's capacity for control as he valued his own security.

One day, after a week's leave of absence, I set about my routine round of this ward by entering through the back door leading into the verandah. The beds were all of them unoccupied, and when I found Charge Nurse Jim he simply remarked, quite casually, 'By the way, the verandah's empty now during the day. I just decided to get them all up.'

Just like that. Conceivably, Donald Mack had had a fit of progressive patient care and had made the suggestion himself, but I rather think not. This quiet, unobtrusive approach to the improvement of people's lot seemed to be the hallmark of the best of care among long-stay patients. One saw it again and again.

Years later, yet another Jim (let's call him Jim Theard) showed a marked contrast to Jim Two's approach.

Jim Theard was a tall, gangling man, dour, taciturn and disenchanted. He had the charge of what had once been the 'refractory ward', and by now had become, with the advent of sundry tranquillisers and anticonvulsants, one of the more interesting wards of the hospital. Jim Theard did not see it like that at all. For my part, the variety of people on the ward was stimulating in itself. All of them were young enough and vigorous enough to show some kind of promise as well as demanding rather more than the kind of simple custodial care (and I do mean care) which allowed the charge to occupy his office most of the day and to run his ward by the simple expedient of raising his voice a little as occasion demanded. (In the male admission ward at Bishopsgate, in the days when it was usual to keep newly admitted patients in bed for a minimum of one week, the hospital had had a charge nurse who knew the creak of every bed individually, and could almost run the ward without sight of it: he was known to sit at his desk, with his back to the door, and call out to his staff, 'Hey, Bob, Mclaren's gettin' oot o' his bed.')

But to return to Jim Theard, it seemed to me that his work was a specialised and valuable one within the context of the hospital, for without it everybody else would have had to exercise a slightly more oppressive regime which could have reflected on the general standard of care everywhere. Yet Jim Theard could not see his work by any means as a specially skilled, valuable or challenging opportunity. In his eyes, he ran a dead end, a place for people that nobody else wanted, and in the end, this vision of his mission in life came to oppress him so much that he took early retirement (and quite clearly benefited from it).

Yet more than this, Theard saw his staff through the same jaundiced veil that coloured his vision of the working day. He spoke rarely, and then tersely, bottling up his feelings behind a tense, florid countenance. But one day, as we happened to pass the large notice-board in his office, he jerked a thumb contemptuously in the direction of the staff timetable.

'And would you look at what I've got to work with!'

Any suggestion from his senior staff was always met with some morose objection, and the physical arrangement of the ward, as well as the structure of the working day, remained as though set in concrete.

And yet, and yet.

Jim Theard had some 30 individuals under his care, all of them lively, and some unpredictable. Among them were two for whose chances I would not have given very much.

One of these was a native Icelander, somehow caught up in the turbulence of the war and spewed up in our remote corner of our own island. His English was fragmentary, and I took him, perhaps mistakenly, to be a schizophrenic of the variety known as 'simple' (the term in this case not implying anything about his intelligence). He approached me on one occasion to discuss the possibility of visiting friends or relatives in Denmark who had written to him and invited him to go to see them. His English was quite adequate to this situation, and he produced the relevant letters in support of his request. There could have been no objection to him going to Denmark, but he was stateless, and I could not imagine that he would be able to find the fare for his journey.

Neither objection held any water. He had, entirely on his own initiative, determined the procedures appropriate to stateless people, and he had been saving up his pocket money diligently for months on end to meet the fare, the amount of which he was quite familiar with. He was a softly spoken individual, and I simply made a note of his plans without for a moment imagining that anything could come of them.

But I was wrong. Jim Theard approached me a little later and put it to me that if I were agreeable, this man could be employed at a modest rate of pay to undertake some routine work in another part of the hospital, and so pursue his plans for going abroad. I was inclined to demur and make light of the idea, but big, surly, taciturn Jim sat himself down and expounded at length, quietly, slowly and very clearly, upon the man's extraordinary determination in pursuing the intricacies of his proposal, and upon the dedication with which he had accumulated a sizeable proportion of the amount of money he needed. Surely, he put it to me, such painstaking resolution deserved to be encouraged.

Obviously, Jim's judgement was correct, and his ideas were put into action. Shortly afterwards there was a wholesale reorganisation of the ward, and I lost touch with the man concerned, but I have no reason to doubt that everything went swimmingly, and that Peter Petersson was duly reunited with his cousins in Denmark.

The other man on whose behalf Jim Theard intervened was an unbecoming character, frankly difficult to like, or even, for that matter, to have much respect for. He had suffered a tiny degree of brain injury at birth which left him prone to occasional convulsions, easily controlled by drugs, but more seriously, prone to peculiarities of his personality which had at one time made him impossible to live with. He had been in the hospital for 20 years or more, and at times he had had occasion to feel the harsher edges of nursing discipline. When I knew him first, all this was in the past, and he was simply a man in late middle age who displayed a certain persistent slovenliness about his person and a curious flat, monotonous way of speaking which made him profoundly uninteresting to talk to. He had either mellowed with age or, with the passage of time, had learned to fit in, and he was no longer a problem to anybody at all. Jim Theard, who might have been glad simply to carry a passenger or to have one of his beds conveniently blocked, was, however, not content.

He put it to me in his own gruff way that Gordon deserved a move towards a more liberal regime. 'After all,' he said, 'the chap deserves it.'

Theard was much better versed than I in the conventions of long-term care, and I could see the force of his argument. Gordon was duly moved to a much quieter and less regimented unit close by. For a while I lost touch with him then, but a year later he turned up in an out-patient clinic at a wan little seaside resort an hour's drive away. Some diligent social worker or a senior nursing officer had dutifully secured his discharge to an erstwhile boarding-house where the proprietrix was glad to have her beds filled on a permanent basis.

Gordon was content in his own pedestrian way, and it was quite enough to see him two or three times a year as a matter of routine. After another year in his new life, he maundered on in his own peculiar way until it turned out that he had taken a fancy for a package holiday to the Hebrides. He showed no great excitement at the prospect, and no special motive for his journey, and for my part I thought no more about it. But at his next visit, he had indeed taken his holiday, and while he had made no special friends during his fortnight, and brought back no particular memories to enthuse about, it was plain that he was, quite naturally, rather proud of his achievement.

Six months later, he came up with the idea that he might fancy a tour on the Continent. He was a bit vague about it and showed no particularly realistic ideas on the subject, and once again I thought no more of it. Yet he turned up six months later and reported on his fortnight in the Low Countries. He was able to tell me which countries he had visited, but not a great deal else, yet he obviously derived a great deal of satisfaction from his new-found independence. In his own small way, he clearly represented a minor triumph for the burgeoning ideals of what came to be called 'community care'. And this could not have come about but for the intervention of a gruff, taciturn man who could by no means be seen as an ideal of patient understanding.

Both of these Jims, of course, have been recalled for a purpose. The fact is that for a full generation, it has become fashionable to peddle the image of institutional care along the lines of *The Snake Pit* (all locked doors and airing courts), assisted by a few smart sociologists and theorists of social administration with everything to gain in academic terms and nothing to contribute in terms of practical responsibility.

It is now unlikely that any accurate and compelling account of the social history of psychiatric nursing will ever become available. The best accounts are scarce and obscure. Certainly the quality of care for the poor and deranged must have varied both between hospitals and within hospitals. Within living memory, the care of the syphilitic, the tuberculous and the 'elderly mentally infirm' has been both unrewarding and demanding, and each of them contributed a significant proportion of the work of the psychiatric nurse.

Neither of our two Jims was in any position to work miracles, yet acquaintance with them, and with countless others of their kind, does suggest that against the impossible social, economic and clinical background of the age, there was available a body of potential goodwill and practical working skill which has been too consistently neglected. Righteous denunciation of all that the old asylums stood for is altogether too glib, and a better perspective, could we but find it, is long overdue.

For the present, another couple of anecdotes must suffice.

When the time came that I was no longer able to serve the community at large, one man insisted that he would see no one but myself, and I was able to find a small private room where I could see him occasionally until he too changed his occupation and left the area. He was a graduate professional man who had suffered a number of attacks of crippling depression with agitation which apparently left him practically incoherent. He had spent periods in a number of different institutions over the entire length of the kingdom: fortunately, when I saw him, the worst was past; he had secured a rewarding steady position in his working life, and had acquired a reasonably stable family background to boot.

Basically he required little more than his share of patient attention, together, it must be said, with very small amounts of standard medication which needed to be kept an eye on from time to time. As we got to know each other, he began to relax, and one day before he took off he recalled all the various places where he had been cared for, and then, after an interval for reflection, he launched into an impassioned account of the experience which had affected him the most. This, rather surprisingly, had occurred in a very large teaching hospital, where he had one day begun to conduct himself in a rather disorderly fashion.

Speaking with great emphasis, in measured, deliberate phrases, he gave me a long account of the situation. A charge nurse and a nursing sister had cajoled him into a hot bath, and had then, turn by turn, sat on the edge of the bath and talked to him by the hour. He recalled both their names, and as he spoke of them, it was clear that he lived again the time that they had spent with him.

Each of them had put to him their understanding that out there on the ward there were many who could not help themselves: people, perhaps, who might be noisy, morose, restless, preoccupied or incoherent. But you, John, they said, have it in you to take charge of your insecurity, your anxieties and your fears. They understood; it would take time for him to come to terms with his situation, but a man of his qualities need not be dominated by them ... and so they spoke to him, gently, candidly, honestly and at great length. He nodded to himself as he relived their patience and their evident understanding, as if to confirm that yes indeed, that was how it had been.

At the end of his account, he reaffirmed that of all his encounters, this one had been the most significant and enduring. And at the end he paused, as if to digest the experience afresh. Yes, clearly, that was how it had been.

Purely as a sidelight, it is perhaps worth remarking that 20 years before, a group of sophisticated medical men had spent weeks trying to determine why one of their subjects was invariably calmer and more lucid on one particular day each week. It turned out that that day was bath day.

* * *

If the ordinary devoted mental nurse could endure unthinkable conditions in the name of society at large, and still retain enough resources to care consistently, and even perhaps sometimes to facilitate the cure of people who could not care for themselves, there were also among them occasional men and women of outstanding qualities which defied categorisation.

Such a one came to us from some centre in Lancashire. So far as I know, no one ever quite discovered exactly where he *did* come from. Quite possibly he had emerged from some small academic unit somewhere; that would have accounted at the same time both for his own reticence on the subject and for his unusually confident and somewhat unorthodox approach to his work.

He took over a busy and potentially difficult ward from the start without any fuss. He announced no plans, inaugurated no new policies, and sublimely ignored any current fashions of work. He was on equally good terms with his staff and patients alike – for Tim, indeed, I could believe they *were* alike. He showed no undue familiarity to any man. His approach to the medical staff was the same. Deference and criticism alike were completely foreign to him. He would inform and he would request, but in all circles he moved so unobtrusively, with such lack of ostentation as to be quite remarkable. In a word, his touch was sure.

I remember him for a particular touch of genius in an especially tricky situation, which perhaps only Tim could have identified. At the time, we had the care of two patients who each in his own way presented idiosyncratic, awkward, intractable problems. Dick, on the one hand, was simply a great, gormless, simple-minded mischief-maker, always out and about, always ready to give a hand, always ready to help – but particularly to help himself. He had an artful way, from time to time, of swindling public bodies into subscribing sums of money for a charitable cause, which always turned out in the event to be his own pocket. This embarrassment could be minimised simply by keeping an eye on the lad, but it was, to say the least, a constant nuisance.

Little Sidney, on the other hand, presented a much more serious problem. He had been cursed from an early age with a rare and bizarre condition which rejoiced in the name of dementia praecoxissima – in his case, a florid form of simple schizophrenia occurring first in childhood. Sidney presented no great problem as long as he was left alone, when he would curl up in a corner and comment on the world in his own high, whining voice. The early onset of his condition meant, of course, that he had never learned to rub along at any level in society, and had nothing to offer in any kind of community. For a little while it seemed that he might fall prey to the habit of repeating outrageously bawdy rhymes, without the least indication of understanding what they meant. Fortunately his tormentor soon tired of that game, but inevitably young

Sidney, still in his teens, graduated to Ruff Ward, where just as inevitably he came at the bottom of such pecking order as there was. There he was frankly a thorough nuisance. Giving him a room of his own made matters worse, since he beat a tattoo on the door in a steady rhythm throughout the day, repeating some phrase or other in his high piping whine the whole time. Sedatives and tranquillisers did little to help Sidney's fellows, and much less Sidney himself, since prolonged sedation and lack of exercise left him prone to bouts of bronchopneumonia, when he would of necessity be moved to the sick ward, which was occupied almost entirely by the elderly.

There, sedatives were replaced by antibiotics, and as little Sidney's physical condition improved, so his nuisance value increased: he would return to Ruff and the whole cycle would start all over again. The situation was ripe with a potential for disaster greater than anyone realised at the time. Mercifully, Timothy identified the problem and on his own initiative he set in motion a solution as dramatically simple as it was effective.

He put young Sidney into the personal charge of the great, gangling, overactive Dick. The two of them could be seen together around the spacious grounds of the hospital at all times. Both were out of mischief. Dick's great moon of a face beamed with pleasure at the trust placed in him, and Sid for his part was at last able to prattle away inconsequentially as he pleased, and to receive the constant undivided attention which his own pathetically inadequate family had been unable to provide. Years later, I saw him out and about in the nearby town in the company of a young nurse. He had acquired enough in the way of social grace to be perfectly acceptable company in public. He could respond appropriately when addressed, and between times he was content to remain silent in his own peculiar ruminative way. Timothy Thompson's perception had been accurate beyond any expectation. If his response had spoken to the most elementary needs of the human being, it was still a stroke of intuitive imagination which far outran any kind of orthodoxy in the general run of nursing practice.

Tim did not stay with us very long, and soon returned for promotion in his own part of the world. We never saw him or heard of him again. It was almost as though he had never been. Of course, he was not unique: men of vision are memorable in any walk of life. It was my good fortune to have known a few, here and there, who saw further than most.

9

Coda

Arthur had come to us through the courts, and I knew of him only through routine visits to his ward. He was a lean, lanky character who never had much to say for himself, but given a modest dose of tranquilliser, he was alert enough, a hard worker, and well liked by all and sundry. Both 'learning difficulties' and schizophrenia ran in the family, and since his voices had induced him to set fire to a farm outhouse somewhere, we were always careful to monitor his drugs and to be well aware of his whereabouts at all times. Apart from his intrinsically likeable nature and his brush with the law, there would have been nothing of general interest to record about him.

It happened, however, that one teatime I was asked to visit his ward before going home; in fact, before I did anything else, in order to have a look at Charlie, who had 'had a collapse' before he could leave the tea table.

When I got there, Charge Nurse explained that Charlie had collapsed quite suddenly after finishing his tea, and had shown no signs of making any recovery. Since the other 30-odd people in the ward had also been still seated at their places, it had seemed best to move Charlie to a side-room, where he lay, still and quiet on a bed. I took care to examine him scrupulously, and in the circumstances I left the room with some sobriety, closed the door gently and went to make an entry in his notes.

On the way, I was approached by Arthur, who apologised

for delaying me, and asked if I could tell him how Charlie was. I told him that I thought all Charlie's troubles were now at an end, and Arthur, who had evidently anticipated the situation, went on to explain that, well, he and Charlie was mates, and he, Arthur, would like to attend Charlie's funeral.

He went on to explain quite clearly and simply that he understood that he was not allowed to leave the grounds of the hospital without the 'Seckertary of State' giving his approval, and he asked if I might take what steps I could to get this done.

The funeral was a full week away, and the Seckertary of State's approval for Arthur's absence turned out to be something of a formality.

The funeral was to be held in a public cemetery not far away, and on the appointed day we all trooped off to the bare little chapel in the grounds. The hospital chaplain said a few words, a few brief decencies were observed, and then we all trooped off again on foot towards Charlie's grave. Since Charlie was a pauper, he was to be buried in a field just beyond the cemetery itself, which lay in gently rising ground bounded at the far end by the wide open space of a large common.

The day was sunny and mild, yet as we passed the fence which bounded the cemetery proper, a gentle gust of northerly air caught us, and I shivered involuntarily. At this the charge nurse (Bill, it was) caught my eye.

'Aye,' he said, in a half-jesting little undertone, 'it aye blows a bit keener, this corner of the ground.'

In the whole sizeable field there was no headstone, no memorial at all to those who lay there. Years later, among the hospital records I came across a single sheet of paper with their names written in by hand, three to each plot. It seemed then a bitter little memorial, well suited to the sharp breeze which I had thought to feel as we paid homage to Arthur's mate.

It was, of course, Arthur's breathtaking dignity and composure which prompted my remembrance of this whole episode. If the bleak anonymity of Charlie's fate made a chilling symbol of all our ends, it was the dignity and composure of his friend which had led me to that scene.

The farthest journey I had ever made had taken me to O'Hare Field in Chicago, where a nameless uniformed American – a guardian at the gate – had divined the purpose of a different kind of journey. Arthur, as well as his kindred spirit at Bishopsgate, who brought my thinking to a stop when I met them, may as well do so now.

After all, are not those who go to peer down a well likely to see no more than a faint distant image of their own face?

REFERENCES

1 (p.x) ANDERSON, R, 'A Psychoanalytic Approach', *British Medical Journal* vol. 300, 1990, p. 1262.

2 (p.27) HENDERSON, D K & GILLESPIE, R D, *Text-Book of Psychiatry*, Oxford University Press, 1940.

3 (p.28) ibid.

4 (p.32) FOX, T F (ed.), *In the Mental Hospital*, Lancet publications, 1958.

5 (p.70) FRASER, D (ed.), *The Christian Watt Papers*, Caledonian Press, 1988.

6 (p.80) FREEMAN, H, 'Conversation with Robert Cawley', *Psychiatric Bulletin* No. 14, 1993, p. 265.

7 (p.81) PORTER, R, *Mind-Forg'd Manacles*, Penguin, 1990, p. 135.

8 (p.82) FRASER, D (ed.), *The Christian Watt Papers*.

9 (p.92) PORTER, R, *Mind-Forg'd Manacles*.

10 (p.92) HENDERSON, D K & GILLESPIE, R D, *Text-Book of Psychiatry*.

11 (p.92) WOODS, E A & CARLSON, E T, 'The Psychiatry of Pinel', *Bulletin of the History of Medicine* vol. 35, 1981, p. 22.

12 (p.97) NORRIS, C. *Derrida*, Fontana, 1987, p97.

13 (p.112) ALLDERIDGE, P, 'Hospitals, madhouses & asylums: cycles in the care of the insane', in R M Murray and T H Turner (eds.), *Lectures on the History of Psychiatry*, Gaskell, 1990.

14 (p.113) RUSSELL, R, 'The lunacy profession and its staff in the nineteenth century', in W F Bynum, R Porter & M Shepherd (eds.), *The Anatomy of Madness*, Vol. III, Routledge, 1988.

15 (p.113) MACDONALD, K, 'Keepers to Carers', in J Andrews and I Smith (eds.), *Let There Be Light Again*, Greater Glasgow Health Board, 1993.

RECOMMENDED ADDITIONAL READING

Crammer J. *Asylum History* Gaskell, London 1990.